RADIANT SKINCARE - YOUR PATH TO GLOW

The Key to Great Skin is within Your Power - Your Reach

MechieBee

MechieBee

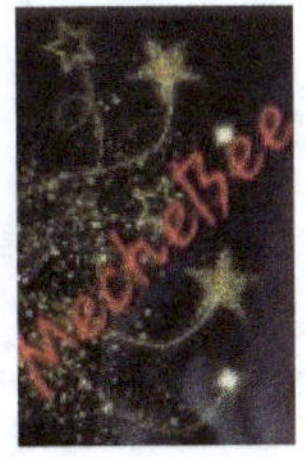

CONTENTS

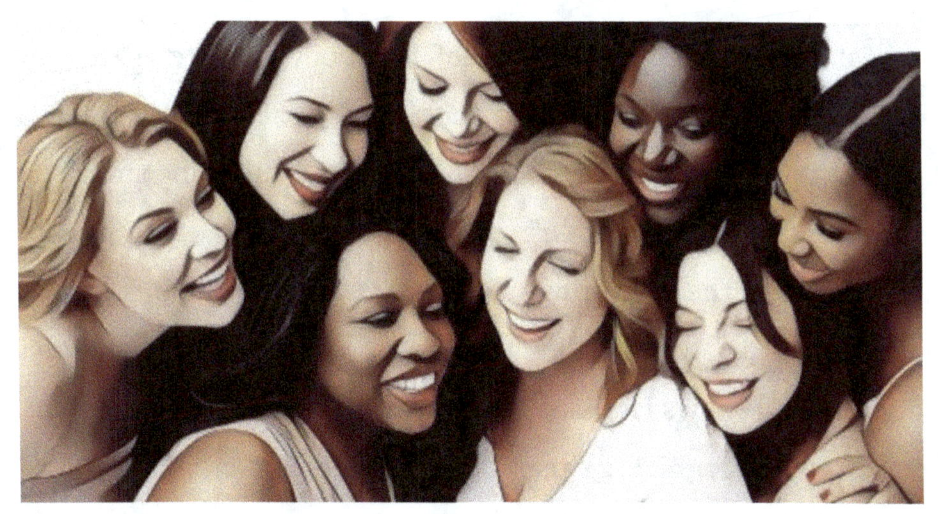

INTRODUCTION

*The Key to Great Skin is within
Your Power – Your Reach*

In a world teeming with beauty advice, quick fixes, and overnight miracles, navigating the path to resolving stubborn facial skin problems can feel like an insurmountable task. Yet, the journey to understanding and caring for your skin is a deeply personal and rewarding endeavor. This e-book is crafted to be your companion through this journey, offering quick, effective, and direct solutions to the skin challenges many women face daily.

Our skin, the largest organ of our body, is a reflection of our overall health, emotions, and life experiences. It's always important to remember that our skin is no different than our moods. Each day may require a different approach, adapting to its current state, the environment, and our overall wellbeing. Just as our moods can shift from joy to sadness, or from calm to anxiety, our skin too shows its discontent through breakouts, dryness, or sensitivity. Recognizing this intimate connection emphasizes the importance of not just knowing but understanding our skin.

Knowing thy skin is no different and as important as knowing thyself, regardless of skin type. This knowledge isn't just about identifying whether you have oily, dry, or combination skin. It's about understanding how your skin reacts to stress, hormonal changes, environmental factors, and different products. It's about listening to your skin and responding with love, care, and patience.

Of course, there are certain skin concerns that remain consistently intertwined with behavioral and/or physiological traits. For instance, the location of acne on your face isn't just a random pattern; it usually is a blueprint. It can be highly informative, offering clues about underlying causes and guiding us towards more effective solutions. For example, acne on the forehead might suggest lifestyle stressors or digestive issues, while breakouts along the jawline often point to hormonal imbalances.

This e-book will guide you through identifying your skin's unique needs, understanding the root causes of common skin problems, and providing adaptable solutions tailored to those issues. From acne to hyperpigmentation, from sensitivity to the signs of aging, we will explore a range of topics with practical advice and recommendations. Our goal is not just to treat skin problems but to foster a relationship with your skin that is based on understanding, respect, and nurturing.

While I am not a licensed dermatologist, my experience and knowledge in skincare allow me to offer valuable insights and guidance to individuals seeking assistance with their skin concerns. Over years of study and research, I have gained a profound understanding of skincare principles, ingredients, and practices, enabling me to provide informed recommendations and solutions. By staying abreast of old and updated developments in skincare science and trends, I strive to offer accurate and reliable information to help others achieve healthier, happier skin. While it's important to consult with a licensed dermatologist for serious or persistent skin issues, I am here to offer support, advice, and encouragement on the journey to better skin health.

Together, we will embark on a transformative journey towards achieving the radiant, healthy skin you deserve. Let's begin this voyage with an open mind and a willing heart, ready 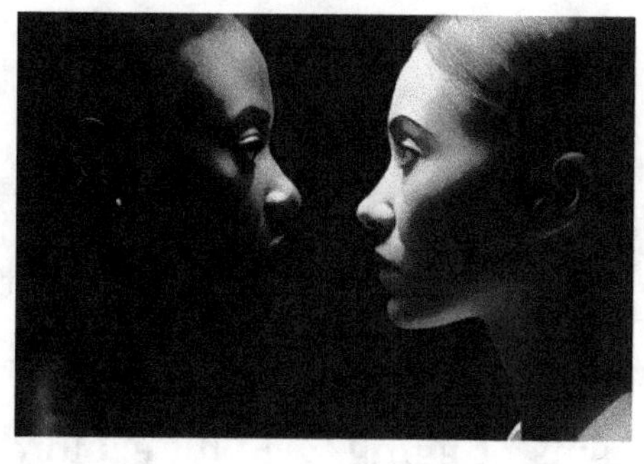 to unlock the secrets of our skin and embrace the beauty of effective, personalized skincare.

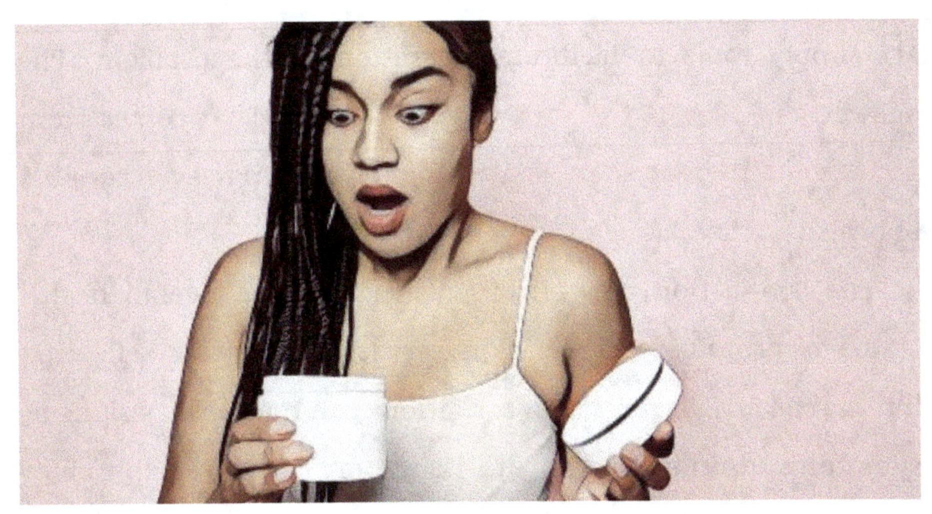

CHAPTER I: THE UNVARNISHED TRUTH ABOUT SKIN CARE

Let's cut straight to the chase: the world of skincare is muddied with myths, marketing ploys, and miracle promises that rarely deliver. Your journey to conquering stubborn facial skin problems won't be found in a fancy bottle or a luxury brand's latest line. The real deal? It's about understanding your skin, its needs, and the science behind what actually works. Skin problems are symptoms. The products that are used are simply tools to facilitate reparation of the problem. The answer **you seek is the root of the problem**. That comes from **understanding why there is a problem** which may even connect to health status.

The connection between skin problems and overall health status is profound, as the skin serves as a mirror reflecting internal health. Various skin conditions can manifest as signs or symptoms of underlying health issues, providing valuable clues for diagnosis and treatment. For instance, hormonal imbalances may trigger acne breakouts, while systemic conditions like diabetes or autoimmune diseases can lead to skin manifestations such as dryness, rashes, or discoloration. Additionally, factors like stress, nutrition, hydration, and lifestyle habits can influence skin health, further emphasizing the intricate relationship between the body's internal well-being and the condition of the skin. Therefore, addressing skin problems often involves not only topical treatments but also addressing underlying health concerns to achieve comprehensive and holistic care.

Always be open to discovering a new path to an old problem. Sometimes, the solutions we've been searching for are wrapped in simplicity rather than complexity. And sometimes, what seems new is quite old.

Identifying Your Skin Type

First, what's your skin type? Determining your skin type is crucial as it dictates the products and treatments best suited for your skin's needs. If you're like me, your answer is probably framed with uncertainty. If so, follow these simple steps to identify your skin type:

1. **Morning Observation: Start by observing your skin in the morning before applying any products. Note its texture, hydration level, and any visible concerns like shine or dry patches.**

2. **Cleansing Test: Wash your face with a gentle cleanser and pat it dry. Wait for about an hour without applying any products.**
    - **Normal Skin: If your skin feels balanced, neither too oily nor too dry, and shows no signs of tightness or discomfort, you likely have normal skin.**
    - **Oily Skin: If your skin feels oily, particularly in the T-zone (forehead, nose, and chin), and appears shiny, you likely have oily skin.**
    - **Dry Skin: If your skin feels tight, rough, or flaky, and lacks moisture, you likely have dry skin.**
    - **Combination Skin: If your T-zone feels oily while your cheeks feel dry or normal, you likely have combination skin.**
    - **Sensitive Skin: If your skin feels irritated, itchy, or reacts easily to products or environmental factors, you likely have sensitive skin.**

3. **Touch Test: Gently touch your skin to assess its**

texture and hydration level.

- **Normal Skin: Feels smooth, soft, and well-balanced.**
- **Oily Skin: Feels slick or greasy, particularly in the T-zone.**
- **Dry Skin: Feels tight, rough, or flaky, especially after cleansing.**
- **Combination Skin: Different areas may feel oily, dry, or normal.**
- **Sensitive Skin: May feel tender, itchy, or inflamed in response to touch.**

By observing how your skin behaves throughout the day and understanding its unique characteristics, you can determine your skin type and make informed decisions when selecting skincare products and treatments. Now skincare warriors, it's time to put your skincare knowledge to the test! Grab a piece of paper, or if you're feeling fancy, fire up your trusty electronic gizmo. Get ready to tackle some questions that'll make your brain cells do the skincare cha-cha-cha! Let's dive in and see how well you know your skin secrets!

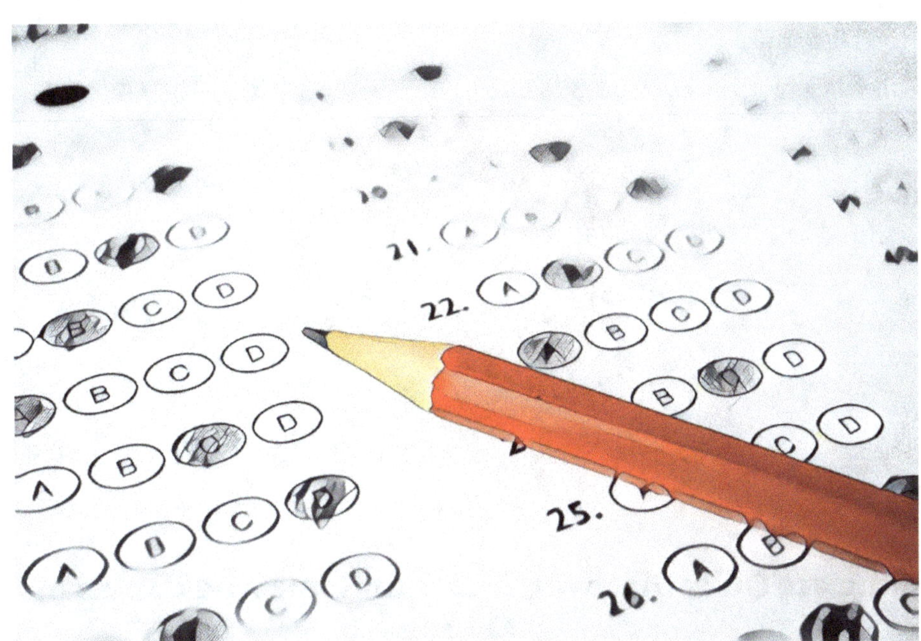

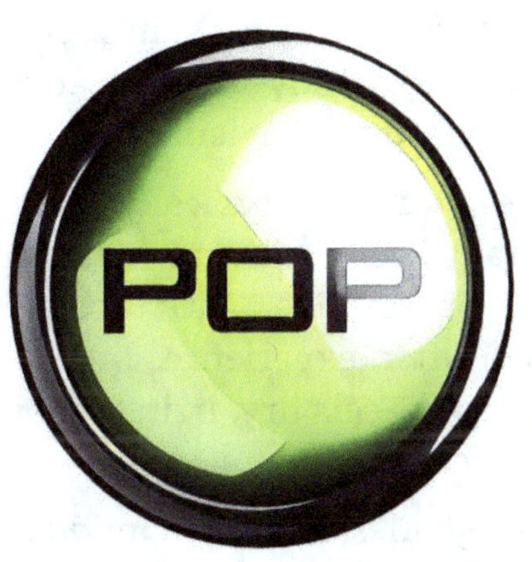
POP

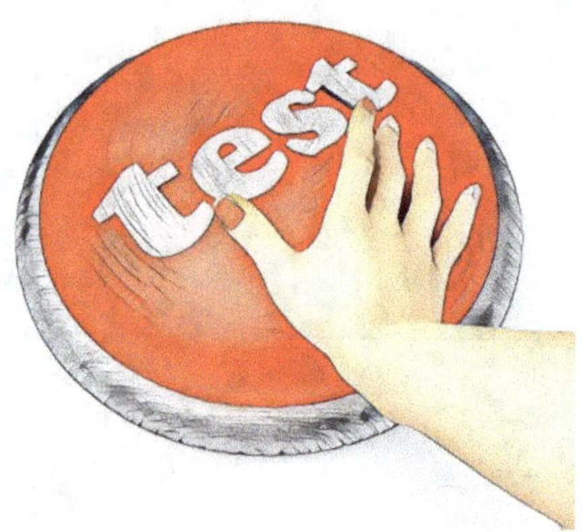

Skincare Quiz: Discover Your Skin Type And Concerns

1. What best describes your skin's texture? a) Smooth and even b) Oily or shiny in some areas, dry in others c) Rough or bumpy with visible pores d) Tight or flaky

2. How does your skin typically react to new products? a) Generally well, with minimal irritation b) Can be sensitive or reactive, with occasional breakouts or redness c) Often experiences breakouts, congestion, or blackheads d) Feels dry, irritated, or itchy after trying new products

3. How does your skin feel by midday? a) Balanced and comfortable b) Oily or greasy c) Dry and tight d) Sensitive or irritated

4. What are your primary skincare concerns? a) Maintaining overall skin health and hydration b) Managing combination skin or occasional breakouts c) Treating acne, blemishes, or congestion d) Addressing dryness, redness, or sensitivity

5. How does your skin typically respond to sun exposure?

a) Tans easily without burning b) Burns occasionally, then tans c) Burns easily and rarely tans d) Sun exposure exacerbates redness, irritation, or dryness

6. Which statement best describes your pores? a) Small and barely visible b) Enlarged or noticeable in the T-zone c) Large and easily clogged d) Tight or invisible, with minimal oil production

7. How does your skin feel after cleansing? a) Clean and refreshed without feeling tight b) Slightly dry or tight in some areas c) Clean but still oily or congested d) Dry, irritated, or stripped of natural oils

Results will be provided in Chapter VI. Happy reading!

Common Skin Problems And Their Causes

As stated in the introduction, "the location of acne on your face isn't just a random pattern; it usually is a blueprint". Here are some quick solutions based on acne location.

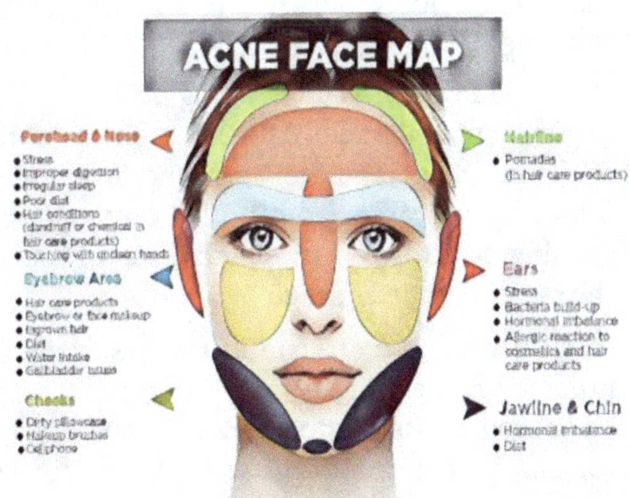

1. **Acne**: Acne occurs when hair follicles become clogged with oil and dead skin cells, leading to the formation of pimples, blackheads, and whiteheads. Hormonal fluctuations, bacterial overgrowth (Propionibacterium acnes), and genetic predisposition are common causes. Hormonal acne often flares up during puberty, menstruation, pregnancy, or menopause. Bacterial acne results from the proliferation of acne-causing bacteria, while cystic acne involves deep, painful cysts under the skin's surface.

➤ **Forehead:** Prioritize stress management and ensure you're getting enough sleep. Consider incorporating digestive aids like probiotics into your diet. Also, ensure your hair products or accessories are not the problem.

➤ **Cheeks:** Evaluate your hygiene practices. Regularly clean your phone, pillowcases, and anything else that frequently touches your face. Pay attention to air quality and consider an air purifier if you live in a polluted area.

➤ **Jawline:** This area often signals hormonal fluctuations. Focus on maintaining a balanced diet and consult with a healthcare provider about potential hormonal treatments or supplements. Some natural treatments for hormonal acne are:

✓ **Evening Primrose Oil:** Evening primrose oil contains gamma-linolenic acid (GLA), an omega-6 fatty acid that may help regulate hormone levels and reduce inflammation associated with hormonal acne. Take evening primrose oil supplements orally according to the recommended dosage.

✓ **Spearmint Tea:** Spearmint tea has anti-androgenic properties, meaning it may help reduce the levels of androgens (male hormones) in the body that can contribute to hormonal acne. Drink one to two cups of spearmint tea daily as part of your skincare routine.

➤ **Nose:** The nose is often affected by enlarged pores and excess oil. Use products with salicylic acid to keep pores clear and manage oil production.

2. **Hyperpigmentation**: Hyperpigmentation refers to dark patches or spots on the skin caused by an excess production of melanin. Sunspots, age spots, and melasma are common forms of hyperpigmentation. Sunspots develop due to prolonged sun exposure. Age spots, or liver spots, are a result of aging and sun damage. Melasma, often triggered by hormonal changes during pregnancy or hormonal therapy, presents as symmetrical patches of darkened skin, typically on the face.

3. **Dryness and Dehydration**: Dryness occurs when the skin lacks sufficient moisture, leading to tightness, flakiness, and rough texture. Dehydration, on the other hand, refers to a lack of water content in the skin. Both conditions can result from environmental factors such as cold weather, low humidity, and excessive sun exposure. Harsh cleansers, hot showers, and certain medications can also contribute to dryness and dehydration.

4. **Sensitivity and Redness**: Sensitive skin is prone to react negatively to external stimuli, such as harsh skincare products, environmental pollutants, and allergens. It may manifest as redness, itching, burning, or stinging sensations. Genetic predisposition, compromised skin barrier function, and underlying skin conditions like rosacea or eczema can contribute to sensitivity and redness. Here's something you may find worthy of dedicated attention. Palmarosa oil has a calming and soothing effect on the skin, which can help reduce inflammation and redness. Palmarosa oil is often touted for its soothing properties and is commonly used in aromatherapy and skincare

products for this purpose. You can comb the internet and see many people reporting positive experiences with using palmarosa oil to alleviate skin irritation, redness, and inflammation. There may not be specific dermatological studies solely focused on palmarosa oil; however, several studies have investigated the potential benefits of essential oils, including those containing palmarosa oil, for skin health. Keep reading to find a DIY recipe in chapter five.

5. **Fine Lines and Wrinkles**: Fine lines and wrinkles are visible signs of aging that occur as collagen and elastin fibers in the skin degrade over time. Factors such as sun exposure, smoking, repetitive facial expressions, and genetic predisposition can accelerate the formation of fine lines and wrinkles. Additionally, intrinsic aging processes, including decreased skin cell turnover and decreased production of natural moisturizing factors, contribute to the development of wrinkles.

Two topical products can serve as an effective and economical way to combat all these skin concerns. They are **rosehip oil** and **DERMA E Vitamin C Concentrated Serum with Hyaluronic Acid**. You can also address these skin issues naturally and internally, taking Methylsulfonylmethane, or MSM for short.

However, I need to address one issue before proceeding – my disclaimer.

*The skincare products suggested in this guide are based on general recommendations and may not be suitable for everyone. It is essential to remember that skincare is highly individual, and what works for one person may not work for another. **<u>Before incorporating any new skincare product into your routine, <u>I strongly recommend</u>**</u>*

<u>performing a patch test. Apply a small amount of the product to a discreet area of your skin, such as the inner forearm, and wait 24 to 48 hours to observe any adverse reactions, such as redness, itching, or irritation.</u>

<u>Furthermore, please consult with a dermatologist or healthcare professional before making significant changes to your skincare routine if you have pre-existing skin conditions, allergies, or sensitivities.</u> They can provide personalized advice tailored to your specific needs and help you choose products that are safe and effective for your skin type.

While I have experienced these products and strive to provide accurate and up-to-date information, the content of this guide is for informational purposes only and should not be considered medical advice. Always use your discretion and seek professional guidance when making decisions about your skincare regimen.

I also want to make this clear: I'm not in cahoots with any of the companies behind the products and tools I recommend. Nope, no secret handshakes or backroom deals here—just me, your friendly neighborhood skincare enthusiast. My face has been exposed to a plethora of products and tools over time which is why I'm recommending these selected ones. They're the cream of the crop, hand-picked by yours truly for their sheer awesomeness. Trust me, I've tried enough to know what's truly valuable in the world of skincare.

And now, let's get back to our regularly scheduled dialogue.

Rosehip Oil

This oil offers numerous benefits for skin health and overall well-being due to its rich composition of vitamins, antioxidants, and essential fatty acids. Some key benefits of rosehip oil include:

1. Moisturization: Rosehip oil is deeply hydrating and nourishing, making it an excellent natural moisturizer for dry or dehydrated skin. It helps restore moisture balance, leaving the skin soft, smooth, and supple.

2. Anti-Aging Properties: Rosehip oil is rich in antioxidants, including vitamin C and vitamin E, which help protect the skin from free radical damage and prevent premature aging. It promotes collagen production, reduces the appearance of fine lines and wrinkles, and improves skin elasticity and firmness.

3. Brightening Effect: The high vitamin C content in rosehip oil helps brighten the complexion and fade dark spots, hyperpigmentation, and acne scars. Regular use of rosehip oil can result in a more even skin tone and a radiant, glowing complexion.

4. Anti-Inflammatory: Rosehip oil has anti-inflammatory properties that help soothe and calm irritated or inflamed skin conditions such as eczema, psoriasis, and rosacea. It reduces redness, swelling, and discomfort, promoting faster healing and relief from skin sensitivity.

5. Scar Healing: Rosehip oil contains essential fatty acids, such as omega-3 and omega-6, which support skin regeneration and repair. It helps fade scars, including surgical scars, stretch marks, and acne scars, by promoting cell turnover and tissue regeneration.

6. Sun Damage Repair: Rosehip oil can help repair sun-damaged skin and protect against further UV damage. Its antioxidant-rich composition helps neutralize free radicals generated by UV exposure, reducing the risk of sunburn, photoaging, and skin cancer.

Overall, **rosehip oil** is a versatile and potent skincare ingredient that offers a wide range of benefits for all skin types. Whether used alone or incorporated into skincare formulations, rosehip oil can help improve skin health, restore radiance, and promote a youthful complexion.

Derma E Vitamin C Concentrated Serum With Hyaluronic Acid

The DERMA E Vitamin C Concentrated Serum with Hyaluronic Acid offers a multitude of benefits for the skin, thanks to its potent blend of ingredients. Here are some of the key benefits:

1. Brightening and Even Skin Tone: Vitamin C is a powerful antioxidant that helps to brighten the skin and fade dark spots, hyperpigmentation, and age spots. Regular use of the serum can result in a more radiant and even skin tone.

2. Collagen Production: Vitamin C stimulates collagen production in the skin, which helps improve elasticity and firmness. This can lead to a smoother and more youthful complexion with reduced fine lines and wrinkles.

3. Hydration: Hyaluronic acid is a humectant that attracts and retains moisture in the skin, providing deep hydration without feeling greasy or heavy. It helps plump and hydrate the skin, leaving it soft, supple, and refreshed.

4. Antioxidant Protection: Vitamin C and hyaluronic acid both have antioxidant properties that help protect the skin from free radical damage caused by environmental

stressors such as UV radiation and pollution. This can help prevent premature aging and keep the skin looking youthful and healthy.

5. Improvement in Texture: The serum helps to improve the overall texture of the skin, making it smoother and more refined. It can also help reduce the appearance of pores, giving the skin a more polished look.

6. Soothing and Calming: The serum contains botanical extracts and other soothing ingredients that help calm and soothe irritated or inflamed skin. This makes it suitable for all skin types, including sensitive and acne-prone skin.

This serum is a versatile skincare product that addresses multiple skin concerns, including dullness, dehydration, aging, and uneven tone. With consistent use, it can help achieve a brighter, smoother, and more youthful-looking complexion.

In fact, a study published in the Journal of Clinical and Aesthetic Dermatology confirmed that vitamin c serum has been found to effectively reduce the appearance of fine lines and wrinkles by promoting collagen production, with study participants experiencing an

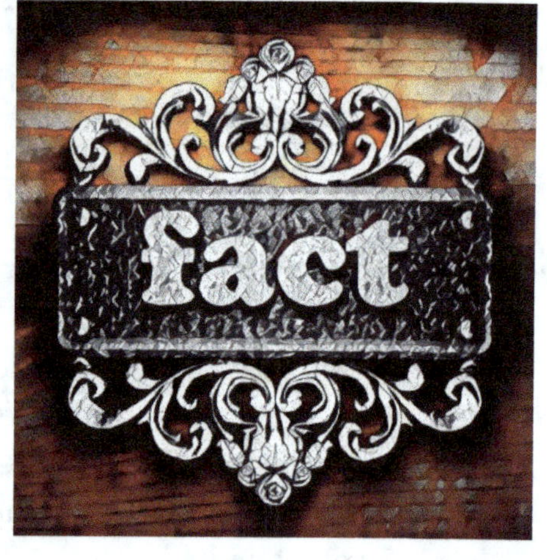

average reduction of 21% of wrinkle depth after twelve weeks of consistent use (www.ncbi.nlm.nih.gov/pmc/articles/

PMC5605218).

What further praises can be sung about these remarkable products? How about this? Individually, each of these products stands as a formidable powerhouse. Yet, when united, they transcend into a realm of sheer extraordinariness, collectively elevating skincare to unparalleled heights. Together, they ignite a skincare revolution, unleashing exceptional, potent, and transformative effects.

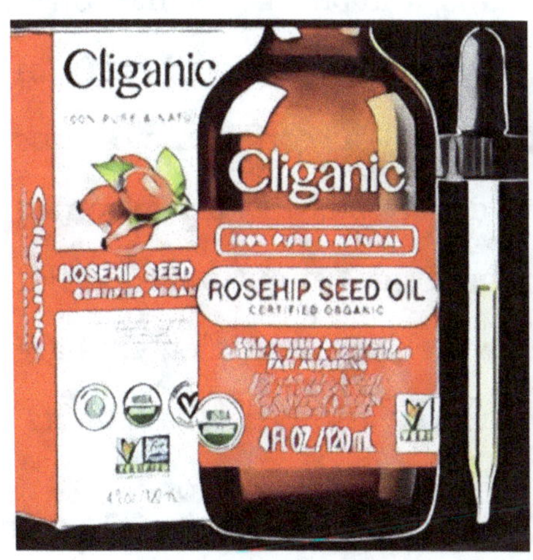

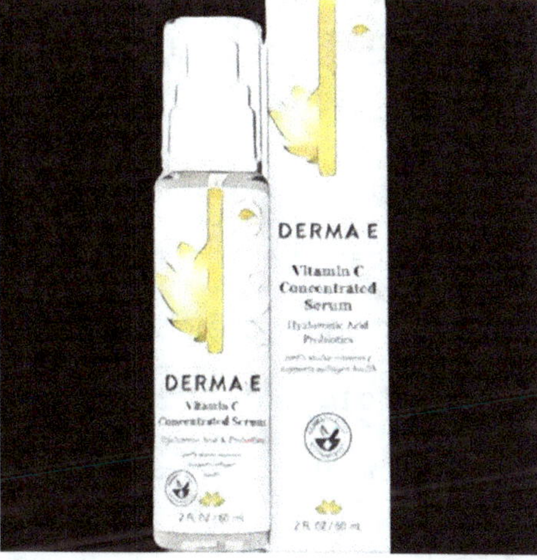

Finally, we come to Methysulfonylmethane or MSM which is well worth mentioning. I can practically hear you saying 'What the heck is MSM?' Well, fret not my curious friend, and take a seat at the front of the class because we're about to learn today. MSM is a naturally occurring compound found in plants, animals, and humans. Small amounts of MSM are naturally produced in the body as a byproduct of the sulphur cycle, primarily in the liver. Sulphur is an essential mineral that plays vital roles in various physiological functions, including protein synthesis, enzyme activity, and the formation of connective tissues.

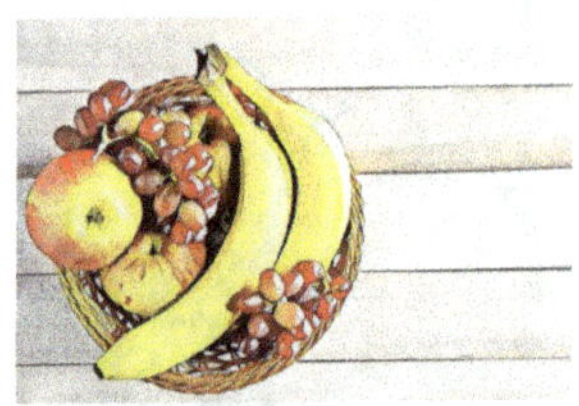

Dietary sources, such as certain fruits, vegetables, grains, and beverages like coffee and tea, are the primary contributors of MSM intake. Before you coffee aficionados gear up for a java jamboree, I have to deliver possibly unwelcomed news. Those dietary sources and beverages mentioned earlier only pack a tiny punch of MSM. However, MSM supplements are available to provide additional support for various health benefits, including joint health, skin health, and immune function.

MSM has powerful anti-inflammatory properties beneficial for skin health. By inhibiting inflammatory pathways and modulating cytokines, MSM helps reduce redness, swelling, and irritation associated with skin conditions like acne, eczema, and psoriasis. It soothes discomfort and itching, promoting overall skin comfort and balance. In case you're wondering what cytokines are and their importance, they are small proteins secreted by various cells in the immune system and other tissues. They act as signaling molecules, regulating immune responses, inflammation, and communication between cells. Cytokines play crucial roles in coordinating the body's response to infection, injury, and disease. In the context of skin health, cytokines are involved in processes such as wound healing, tissue repair, and immune defense against pathogens. However, dysregulation of cytokine production can contribute to inflammatory skin conditions like acne.

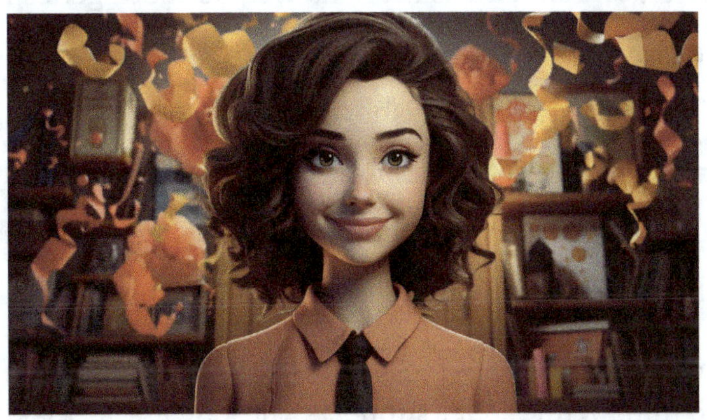

Hey there, still with me? Well, buckle up buttercup because we've just scratched the surface of MSM's superhero abilities. We already know it's a power hitter against acne, sensitivity, and redness, but hold on to your seat because there's more. As a sulphur containing compound, MSM plays a role in collagen synthesis, which can contribute to improved skin hydration and elasticity, potentially reducing dryness. Additionally, MSM may help regulate melanin production, which could lead to a reduction in hyperpigmentation or uneven skin tone over time.

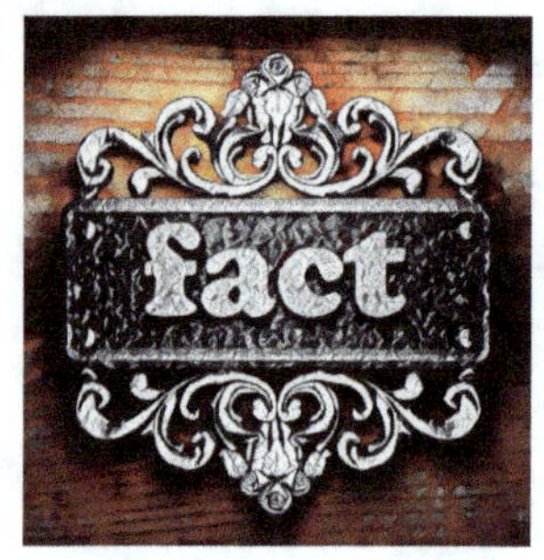

I bring facts again. Even though clinical data is limited, a twelve week study displayed that "oral supplementation with MSM has been shown to influence skin on a genetic level, by regulating a selected number of genes responsible for inflammation, the skin barrier, and moisturisation, as well as those genes involved in the structural integrity of the skin which are associated with the ageing process" (https://shorturl.at/TWZ04). Although, this study involved both collagen and MSM, I believe it's important to highlight that MSM is thought to bolster skin health by stimulating collagen synthesis and enhancing hydration and elasticity in doing so. In other words, MSM and collagen make a dynamic duo. While MSM supports the process in making new collagen protein, molecules, and fibers, collagen provides the skin's structural support. I like to think of it as one ingredient (or two in this case) in the secret sauce of eternal youth.

Are you itching to know what else the study cooked up? Well, I'll tell you friend. "The study's results showed improved dermis density, skin texture, and reduced wrinkles for all active 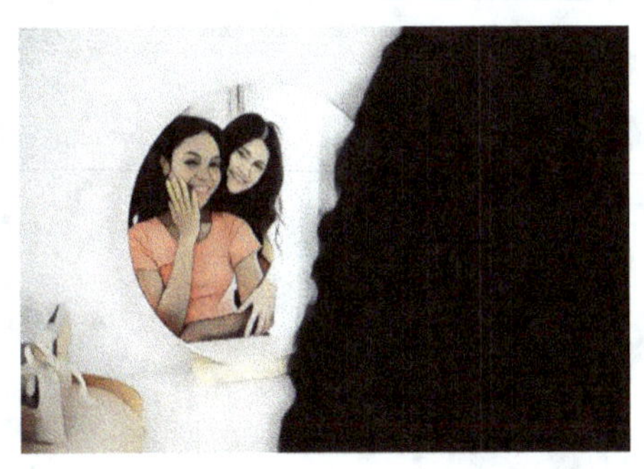 products. However, products containing MSM were superior in improving skin thickness...".

And yes, it's a part of my skin regimen. Although, I must remind you that *individual results may vary, and I'll always advise to consult with a healthcare professional before incorporating any new supplement into your regimen, especially if you have existing health concerns.*

Alright friend, that's a wrap on our MSM crash course for the moment.

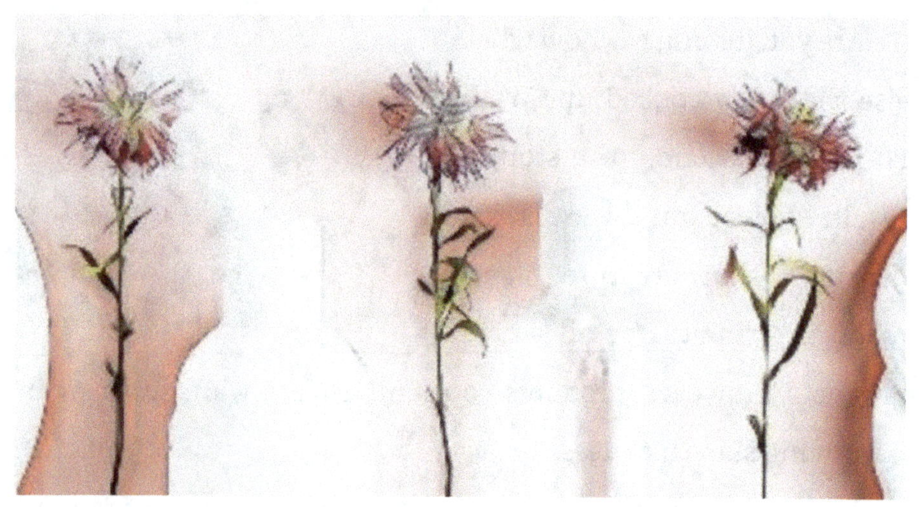

CHAPTER II: BUILDING YOUR SKINCARE ROUTINE

Before you dive into the latest skincare fad or splurge on that expensive serum, let's get something straight: the foundation of good skin health lies in mastering the basics. Cleansing, toning, moisturizing, and protecting your skin from the sun are the cornerstones of any effective skincare routine. If you're not doing these four things right, it's time to reset and refocus. The basics are your best friend: cleansing, toning, moisturizing, and sun protection.

In the canvas of skincare, the basics are the brushstrokes of beauty. Cleansing purifies the canvas. Toning harmonizes its hues. Moisturizing replenishes its vitality, and sunscreen shields its masterpiece from the ravages of time. Together, they weave the tapestry of radiant skin, revealing the true artistry of self-care.

Essentials Of A Daily Skincare Routine

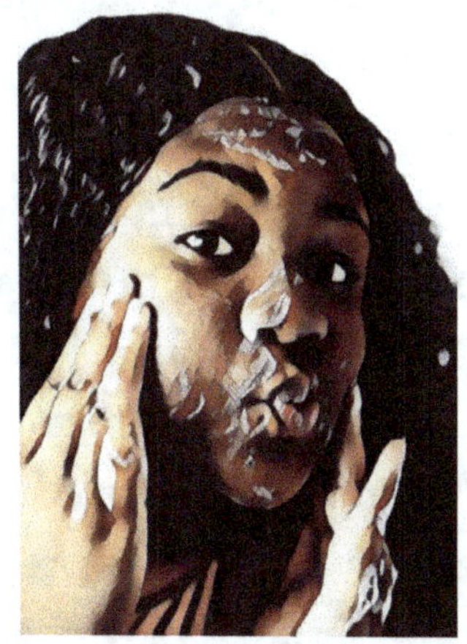

1. **Cleansing:** Opt for a gentle cleanser that doesn't strip your skin of its natural oils. Harsh soaps can do more harm than good, leading to a cycle of dryness and oil overproduction. To cleanse your face like a pro, start by wetting your skin with lukewarm water to open up those pores. Then, apply a dime-sized amount of your favorite gentle cleanser onto your fingertips and massage it onto your face using circular motions. Be sure to focus on areas prone to oiliness or makeup buildup, like the T-zone.

After about 30 seconds of massaging, rinse off the cleanser with lukewarm water and pat your skin dry with a soft towel. Now, you're left with a clean canvas ready for the next step in your skincare routine. And remember, your cleanser ain't no genie in a bottle – you have put in some elbow grease with those fingers of yours to make the magic happen! So, no slapping and dashing —give it a good ole massage before you splash and dash! For a nourishing cleanse, consider products like Glow Recipe Papaya Sorbet Enzyme Cleansing Balm and *Lily Sado Milk & Manuka Ultra Moisture Face Wash.*

These options cleanse effectively while maintaining the skin's hydration and integrity. The cleansing balm removes makeup, dirt, and impurities from the skin while gently exfoliating which prepares the canvas for the main cleanser - like a trusty sidekick setting the stage for the star performer.

2. **Toning**: Incorporating toning into your skincare routine is essential for balancing the skin's pH levels and preparing it for further treatment. *Lancome Tonique Confort* is an excellent choice, infused with moisturizing ingredients to soothe and hydrate while gently refining the skin's texture. Incorporate it after cleansing to ensure your skin is prepped and primed for maximum absorption of serums and moisturizers. Of course, your journey may find another more suited product. The most important thing is to get that balance in check.

3. **Moisturizing:** Don't underestimate the importance of hydration, even if your skin is as oily as a slice of pizza. Investing in a non-comedogenic (say that three times consecutively) moisturizer tailored to your skin type is essential for maintaining skin health. Consistent application of moisturizers like *Aveeno Positively Radiant Daily Moisturizer, Dime Hyaluronic Acid Serum, Glow Recipe Watermelon Niacinamide Dew Drops, and Heritage Store Rosewater & Glycerin* can provide vital hydration, leaving your

skin nourished, balanced, and radiant. Here's a gold nugget for you. Don't leave home without your hydration station, especially when it feels like you're roasting like a marshmallow on a summer's day! My weapon of choice? A spritz of fancy rosewater—it's like a first-class ticket to Dewyville!

4. **Sun Protection:** Sun damage accelerates skin aging and leads to various issues that should be prevented. Applying a broad-spectrum SPF daily is essential for protecting the skin from harmful UV rays. There are no excuses to skip this crucial step. *Elta MD tinted sunscreen* stands out as a recommended product due to its broad-spectrum protection, shielding against both UVA and UVB rays. Additionally, its tinted formula offers light coverage, evening out skin tone and providing a natural glow. Regular use of this sunscreen helps prevent premature aging, sunburn, and other sun-related skin damage, promoting healthier and more youthful-looking skin. Let me say that AGAIN. Listen up, folks: skipping sunscreen is a skincare sin of epic proportions. Trust me, your future self will be sending thank-you cards once you realize the sun's revenge is real!

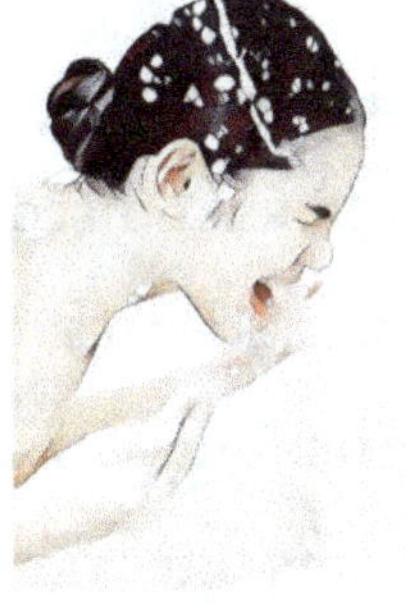

Cleansing is more than just removing impurities. It's self-renewal, washing away the day's burdens to reveal the inherent beauty and resilience within self. In this act of purification, we honor the skin as it reflects the processes of our innermost self. This is

nourishment for both body and soul.

Advanced Skincare Treatments

Exfoliation is key to maintaining healthy skin, but it's essential to choose the right type and frequency for your skin type. *The Peter Thomas Roth Pumpkin Enzyme Mask* is a potent exfoliant that combines physical and chemical exfoliation to reveal smoother, brighter skin. I also love the *Minimo Glow Turmeric Mask.* It is a skincare product formulated to brighten and rejuvenate the skin. Infused with turmeric, a natural ingredient known for its anti-inflammatory and antioxidant properties, this mask helps to reduce the appearance of hyperpigmentation, acne scars, and blemishes, leaving the skin with a radiant glow.

Its gentle exfoliating properties also help to unclog pores and promote smoother, more even-toned skin. I believe it to be suitable for all skin types; however, conduct a patch test before full exposure. And let me tell you, that glow is so bright, it's like my face moonlights as a disco ball after I rinse! Depending on your skin's tolerance, aim to exfoliate 1-3 times per week to avoid irritation and over-exfoliation.

Masks and serums offer targeted solutions to address specific skin concerns. *Naturium Azelaic Topical Acid 10%* and *Naturium Tranexamic Topical Acid 5%* are potent serums that help fade hyperpigmentation and improve overall skin tone. Meanwhile, *Derma E Vitamin C Concentrated Serum* provides antioxidant protection and boosts collagen production, resulting in firmer, more youthful-looking skin. These products are like my trusty sidekicks in my skincare regimen, always ready to lend a hand... or a pump!

Spot treatments are essential for combating breakouts effectively. *Mighty Patch: The Original* is a hydrocolloid patch that absorbs impurities and speeds up the healing process of blemishes. These miniature patches have truly worked wonders for me. I've banished those pesky pimples faster than you can say "abracadabra" with these little rascals! For more stubborn acne, *IL Makiage Power Polish* contains shea butter and jojoba oil spheres. The shea butter moisturizes, and jojoba oil is practically an all-in-one oil. Jojoba oil is hydrating, moisturizing, nutritional (vitamins B & E along with minerals), non-acnegenic, non-allergic, and anti-microbial. If that's not enough, it serves as an exfoliant and is anti-aging. Both ingredients in this polish reduce the appearance of dullness, textures, pores, breakouts, and discoloration.

I wouldn't be a good friend if I didn't say don't underestimate those budget-friendly options, such as *Queen Helene Mint Julep Masque*. This masque aids in deep cleansing, skin purification, pore shrinkage, and refreshes dull complexions with its minty formula. It also serves a a spot treatment by drawing out impurities when placed on the blemish or problem area. This reduces inflammation.

Addressing **delicate areas like the under-eye** requires specialized care. *Oil of Olay Eye Lifting Serum* provides intense hydration and helps reduce the appearance of fine lines and wrinkles around the eyes. 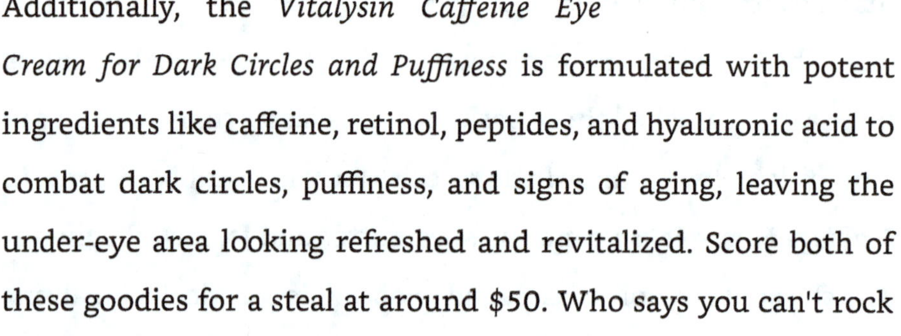 Additionally, the *Vitalysin Caffeine Eye Cream for Dark Circles and Puffiness* is formulated with potent ingredients like caffeine, retinol, peptides, and hyaluronic acid to combat dark circles, puffiness, and signs of aging, leaving the under-eye area looking refreshed and revitalized. Score both of these goodies for a steal at around $50. Who says you can't rock fabulousness on a budget?

In the pursuit of radiant skin, the suggested advanced skincare treatments serve as guiding beacons, illuminating the path to transformation and empowerment, for within their meticulous formulations lie the promise of renewed vitality and timeless beauty.

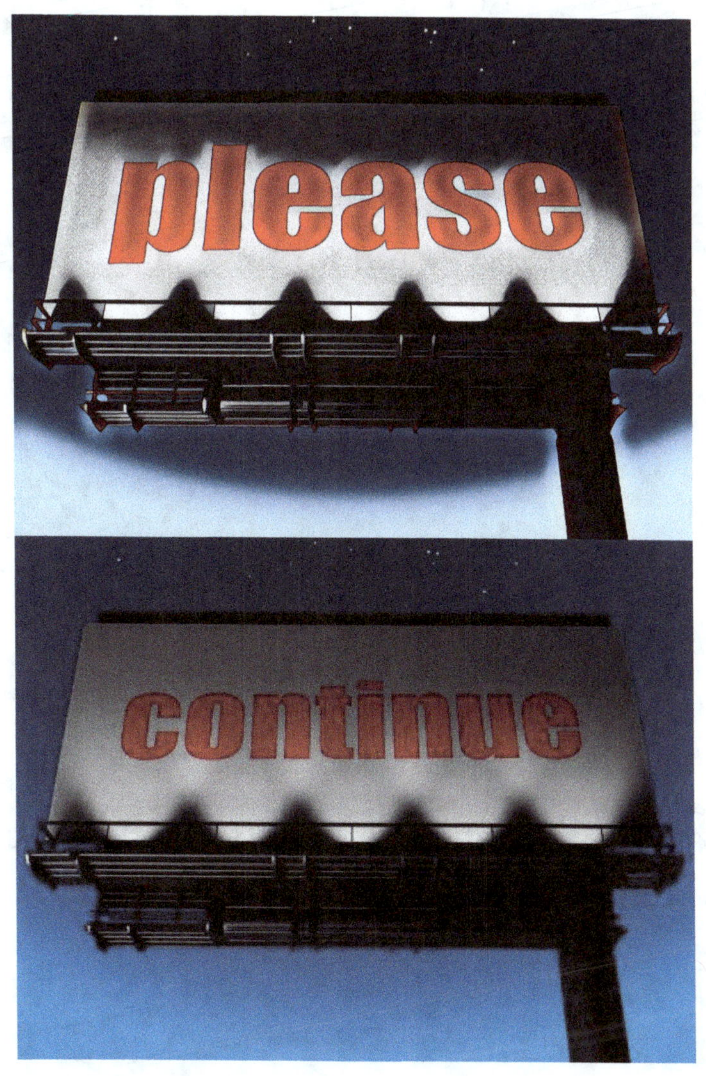
please
continue

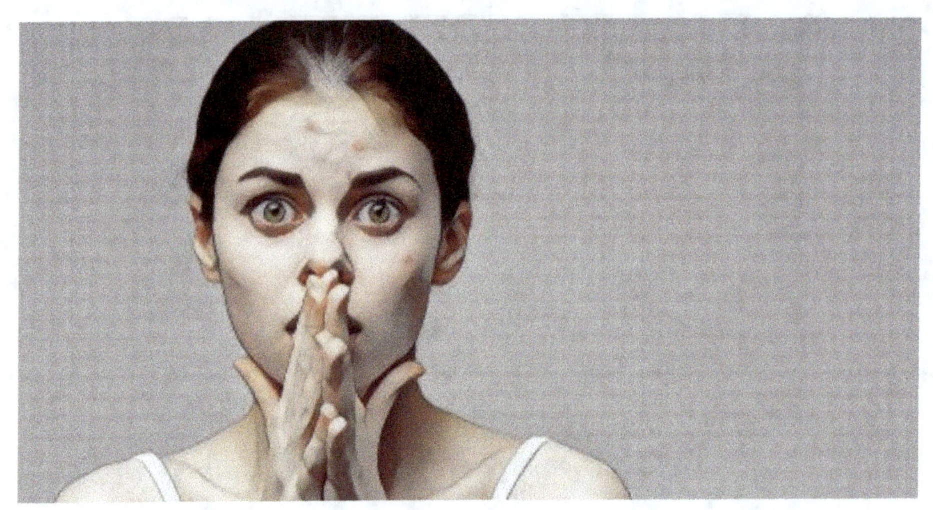

CHAPTER III: SPECIAL FOCUS ON STUBBORN PROBLEMS

Acne Management...

Ah, the bumpy road of acne - it's like having a secret admirer who just won't take a hint! One day you're feeling confident, strutting your stuff, and the next, bam! You wake up with a new friend right smack dab in the middle of your face. It's like your skin is playing a game of whack-a-mole; however, instead of moles, it's pimples popping up to say hello!

And don't even get me started on those stubborn ones that think they're the rulers of your face, refusing to budge no matter what you throw at them. It's like they've taken up permanent residence, complete with a "no vacancy" sign!

Acne can be a persistent challenge, but establishing daily routines is key to prevention and management. Begin with a gentle cleanser like *EltaMD Foaming Facial Cleanser*, which effectively removes impurities without stripping the skin's natural oils. Follow up with a serum like *Naturium Niacinamide Serum 12% Plus Zinc 2%* to regulate oil production and reduce inflammation. For spot treatment, consider using products containing benzoyl peroxide or salicylic acid, such as *Derma E Acne Blemish Control Treatment Serum*. If acne persists or becomes severe, **it's advisable to consult a dermatologist** who can recommend tailored treatment options like prescription medications or professional procedures.

Hyperpigmentation

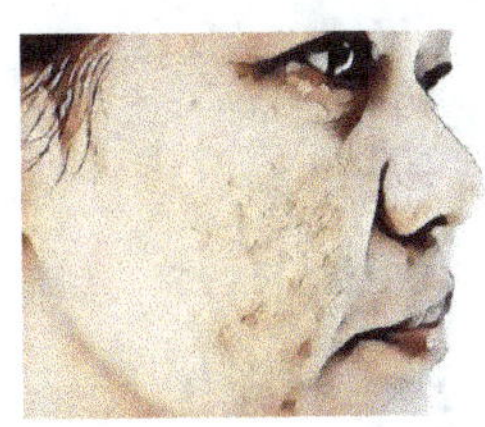

Preventing hyperpigmentation requires diligent sun protection, so be sure to sunscreen like apply *EltaMD UV Clear Broad-Spectrum SPF 46 daily*. Incorporate topical treatments like *Naturium Alpha Arbutin Serum 2%* or *Glow Recipe Watermelon Glow Niacinamide Dew Drops* to target existing pigmentation and inhibit melanin production. For severe cases, professional treatments such as chemical peels or laser therapy may be necessary to achieve significant results. Natural solutions like tea tree oil, castor oil, and rosehip oil can also help lighten dark spots and even out skin tone when used consistently over time. I slather on all these potions and lotions to keep my fabulousness at peak levels (cue the posh accent), and I must say, the results are positively smashing, my darlings!

Sensitivity And Redness

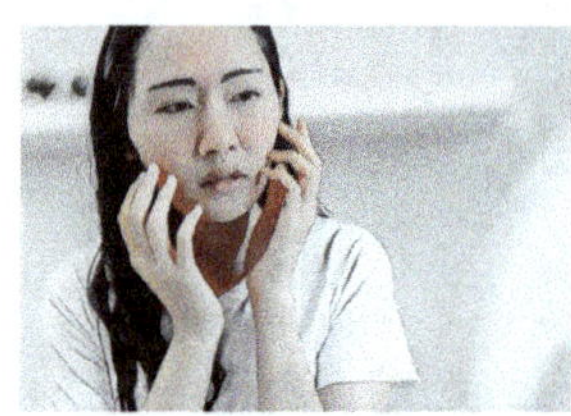

Identifying triggers for sensitivity and redness is essential for effective management. Look for gentle, fragrance-free products like *Derma E Sensitive Skin Cleanser* and *Naturium Plant Ceramide Rich Moisture Cream* to soothe and hydrate sensitive skin. Incorporating natural ingredients such as tea tree oil, known for its anti-inflammatory properties, can help calm irritation and reduce redness. Personally, I'm a fan of *Lily Sado Milk & Manuka Ultra Moisture Face Wash* because it's great for sensitive skin. It's gentle, soothing, and hydrating without any harsh chemicals or fragrances that might throw your skin into a tantrum. Plus, its blend of milk and Manuka honey is like a dream team, leaving your skin feeling as soft as a cloud. **It's very important to know that if sensitivity**

and/or redness persists or worsens, it's advisable to seek professional help. A dermatologist can provide personalized recommendations and prescribe medications like topical corticosteroids or oral antihistamines to alleviate symptoms and improve skin health.

Alrighty friend, I've laid it on thick with the info overload. Now, after bombarding you with all of that, it's time for a pep talk. Ahem..AHEM!!! Fear not, fellow skin warriors for we are resilient! We will do more than master the art of concealing and dabbling with the unpredictability of skincare potions and lotions. We will hone our ninja skills to stop trying to rush the process and/or cover our faces like it's a high-stakes game of operation and the hourglass of sand is nearly empty. We will win this skin battle by being informed, patient, and resilient.

So here's to the ups and downs of skin problems - the unpredictable rollercoaster ride that keeps us on our toes, reminding us that even in our most pimpled, red, and uneven 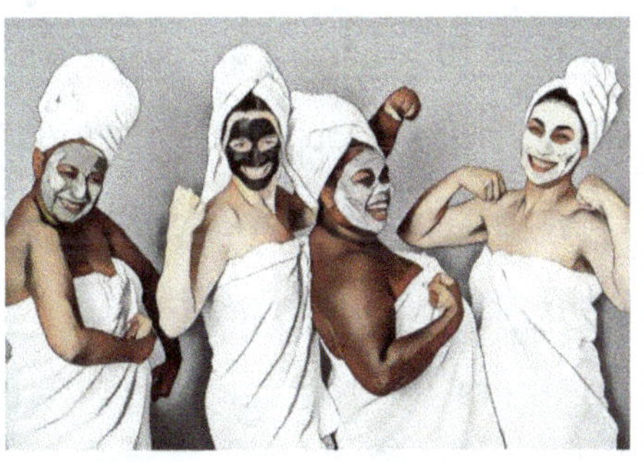 toned moments, we're still fabulous, fierce, and ready to conquer the world, one issue at a time!

Now, let's rev up this knowledge locomotive and get it chugging down the tracks again.

Skincare Tools

I also want to suggest adding these tools into your skincare routine. Skincare tools are like your skin's personal cheerleaders, giving it that extra boost to shine bright like a diamond! From exfoliating brushes to facial rollers, these tools help to remove dead skin cells, promote blood circulation, and enhance product absorption, all while giving you that spa-like pampering you deserve. Think of them as your skin's workout buddies, helping it stay toned, firm, and radiant!

I have purchased so many tools over the past couple of decades. I really like the *Commodery Pore Cleanse Hydration* tool and *Commodery GlowGenie 2.0* tool because they enhance skin cleansing and promote circulation for a radiant complexion.

The *Commodery Pore Cleanse Hydration* tool and *Commodery GlowGenie 2.0* tool are innovative skincare devices designed to enhance your skincare routine and promote healthier, more radiant skin at a fraction of the cost of purchasing bigger brand products in this category. They're also more economical than paying for costly spa treatments. The choice was clear for me. The question I poise to you is **why not have treatments at your fingertips?**

1. *Commodery Pore Cleanse Hydration Tool*: This tool is specifically designed to deep clean pores and hydrate the skin effectively. It utilizes gentle vibrations and

sonic pulsations to dislodge impurities, excess oil, and dead skin cells from deep within the pores, leaving the skin thoroughly cleansed and refreshed. By incorporating the Pore Cleanse Hydration Tool into your skincare routine, you can achieve a deeper level of cleansing that traditional methods may not provide. This can help prevent clogged pores, breakouts, and blackheads, leading to clearer and smoother skin. Moreover, the hydrating function of the tool helps infuse moisture into the skin, leaving it feeling soft, supple, and hydrated after cleansing.

2. ***Commodery GlowGenie 2.0 Tool***: The GlowGenie 2.0 tool is designed to promote circulation and boost the absorption of skincare products, enhancing their effectiveness. It features microcurrent technology that gently stimulates the facial muscles, helping to improve blood flow and lymphatic drainage. This results in a brighter, more youthful complexion with reduced puffiness and improved skin tone. By using the GlowGenie 2.0 tool as part of your skincare routine, you can maximize the benefits of your favorite serums, moisturizers, and treatments. The gentle massaging action helps to ensure that skincare products penetrate deeper into the skin, allowing their active ingredients to work more efficiently. This can lead to improved hydration, increased firmness, and a more radiant complexion over time.

Incorporating both the Commodery Pore Cleanse Hydration tool and Commodery GlowGenie 2.0 tool into your skincare routine can help you achieve cleaner, more hydrated skin with a brighter, more

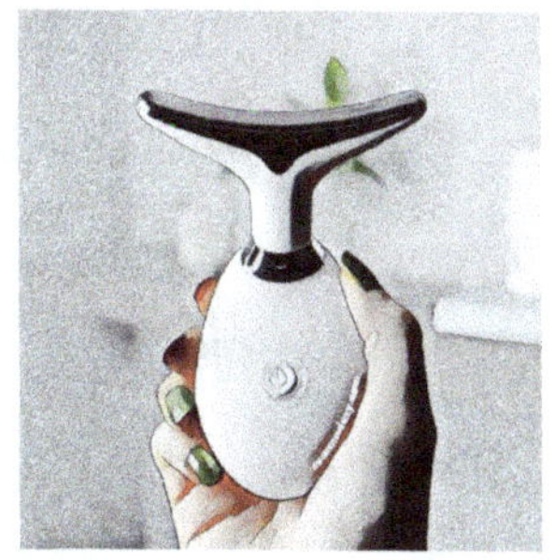

youthful appearance. These devices offer advanced skincare solutions that complement traditional skincare products and techniques, making them valuable additions to any skincare regimen. And yep, I splurged on both. Gotta keep that youthful vibe going strong, like I'm the Peter Pan of skincare!

I also use the Gillette Venus razor for dermaplaning. Prior to using the Gillette razor, I always used various razors to remove my facial hair, and I noticed that it also helped to remove dry skin, leaving my complexion smoother. Surprisingly, I discovered that "dermaplaning" was the term for this technique. Dermaplaning not only removes unwanted hair but also exfoliates the skin, promoting a brighter, smoother, and more radiant complexion.

My other mentions are very strong competitors and elevate the skincare game like the Commodery tools. They are NuFACE and PMD. The NuFACE is a handheld microcurrent device designed for at-home facial toning and contouring. It delivers low-level electrical currents to the skin, stimulating facial muscles to improve tone and reduce the appearance of wrinkles. The PMD skin tool is a handheld device used for at-home skincare treatments. It typically utilizes microdermabrasion and vacuum suction technology to exfoliate the skin, remove dead cells, and promote cell renewal. This improves the skin's texture, tone, and overall appearance, resulting in a smoother in more radiant complexion. Do I have these gadgets? Of course I do friend.

They're definitely worth the dough, but truth be told, I'm a deal hunter extraordinaire! I'll wait for holiday specials, Mother's Day bargains, well, any deal that'll score me the gadget that I'm itching for. After all, why pay full price when you can have the joy of snagging your desire for a sweet deal.

Embrace skincare tools as catalysts for skin transformation, as they elevate skincare treatments to profound experiences of rejuvenation and self-care. Through their gentle touch, these tools transcend the normal skincare routine and become eager, anticipated moments of self-love and empowerment.

The Myth Of The Miracle Cure

If I had a dime for every "miracle cure" that hit the market, I'd be writing this from a yacht. Here's the blunt truth: 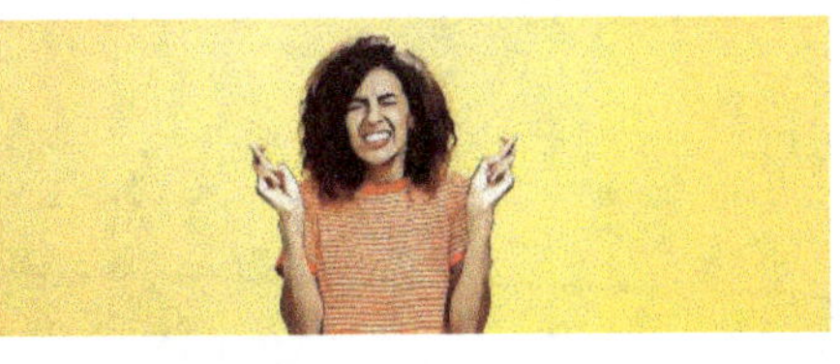 there is no one-size-fits-all solution in skincare. What works miracles for one person might do absolutely nothing for another. Your skin's needs are as unique as your fingerprint. This is where the golden rule comes in: Always be open to discovering a new path to an old problem.

Maybe your acne isn't just about your skin type but your diet, stress levels, or the pillowcase you haven't changed in a fortnight. By the way, those beloved cotton pillowcases may be harboring dustmites that are feasting as you sleep not to mention the creases and wrinkles caused by the rough fibers. You might want to switch it up mate. Be willing to look beyond skincare products and consider lifestyle changes that could make a world of difference. As I initially said, what's new may actually be old. Afterall, there's nothing new under the sun.

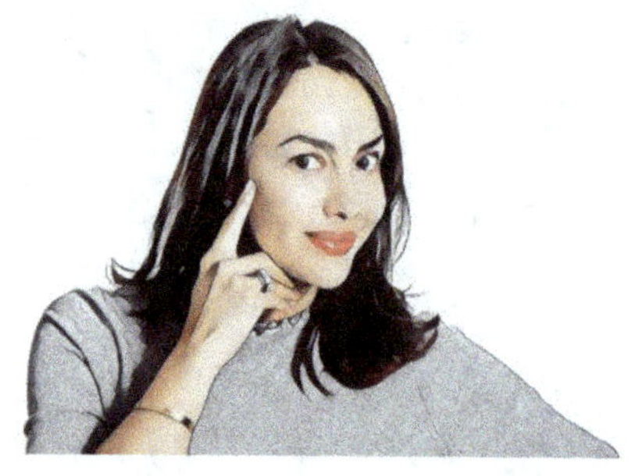

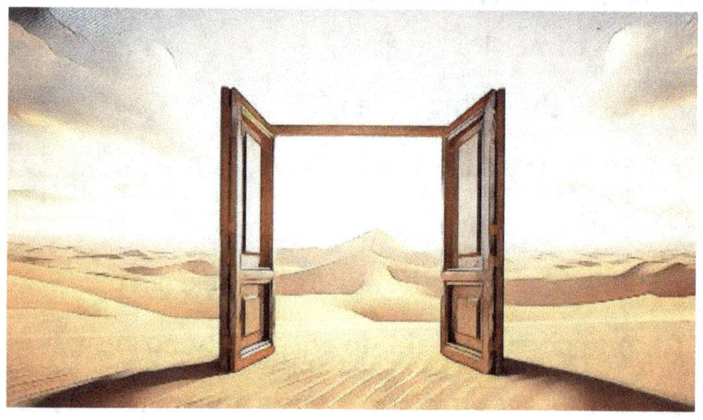

Open-mindedness is the key to unlocking new possibilities and expanding our horizons.

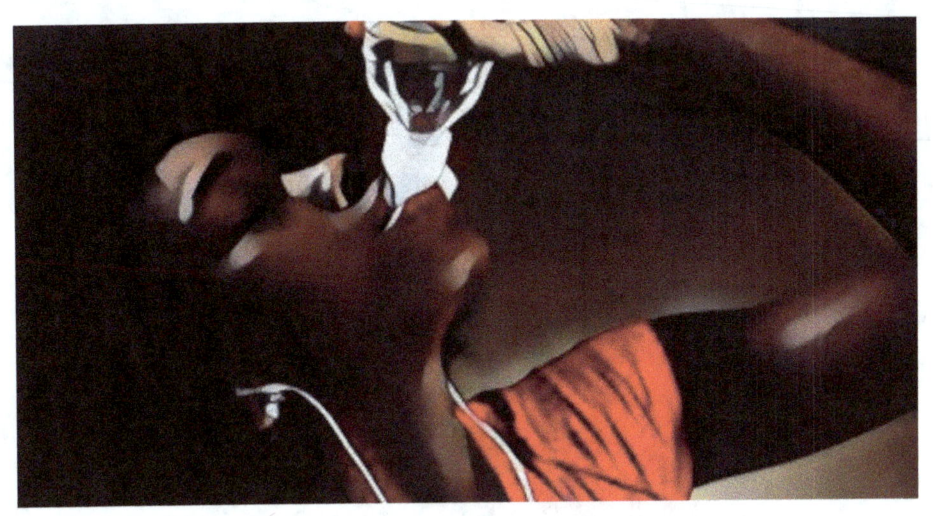

CHAPTER IV: LIFESTYLE AND SKIN HEALTH

Diet and Hydration...

The saying "you are what you eat" holds true when it comes to skin health. Embracing a balanced diet rich in fruits, vegetables, lean proteins, and healthy fats can provide essential nutrients for skin regeneration and repair. Incorporate foods high in antioxidants like berries, spinach, and nuts to combat free radical damage and promote a youthful complexion.

Limiting processed foods, refined sugars, and excessive dairy intake can help reduce inflammation and prevent acne breakouts. Consider incorporating supplements like omega-3 fatty acids, vitamin D, and collagen peptides into your diet to support skin health from the inside out.

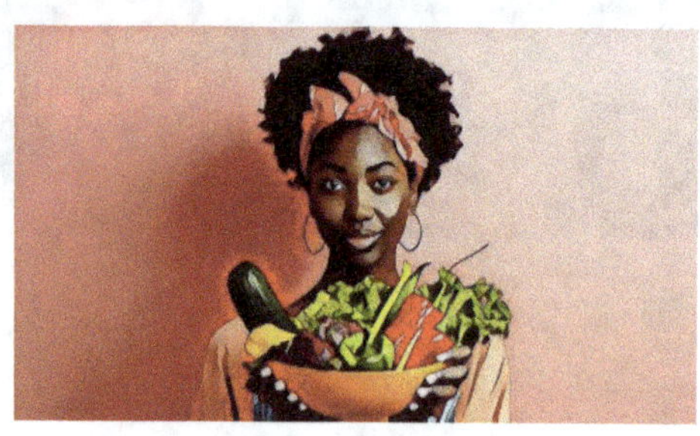

Remember that old adage: garbage in...garbage out!

Staying hydrated is also crucial for maintaining skin health. The human body is composed of approximately 60% water, which plays a crucial role in various physiological functions, including skin health. Water is distributed throughout the body, including within cells, tissues, and organs, contributing to their structure and function. Water is essential for maintaining hydration, elasticity, and overall function. Adequate hydration helps to plump up the skin cells, making the skin appear more youthful and reducing the appearance of fine lines and wrinkles. Water also supports the skin's natural barrier function, helping to protect against environmental stressors, pollutants, and pathogens.

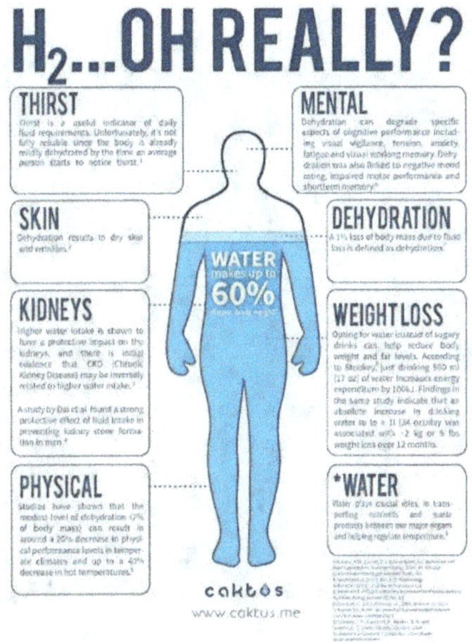

When the body is dehydrated, the skin can become dry, tight, and dull. Dehydration can compromise the skin's barrier function, leading to increased sensitivity, irritation, and inflammation. Chronic dehydration may contribute to various skin issues, including dryness, flakiness, and even exacerbate conditions like eczema and acne. Consuming sufficient water is pivotal for healthy skin as it helps to maintain optimal hydration levels from within. While the exact amount of water needed varies depending on factors such as age, weight, activity level, and climate, a general guideline is to drink at least eight 8-ounce glasses of water per day (the "8x8" rule). Although individual water needs may vary, and it's essential to listen to your body's signals for thirst and adjust your water intake accordingly.

DAILY WATER INTAKE

WEIGHT		8oz/240ml	WATER	
80 lbs	36 kg	5	40 oz	1.2 liter
100 lbs	45 kg	6	50 oz	1.5 liter
120 lbs	54 kg	7	60 oz	1.8 liter
140 lbs	64 kg	9	70 oz	2.1 liter
160 lbs	73 kg	10	80 oz	2.4 liter
180 lbs	82 kg	11	90 oz	2.7 liter
200 lbs	91 kg	13	100 oz	3.0 liter
220 lbs	100 kg	14	110 oz	3.3 liter
240 lbs	109 kg	15	120 oz	3.5 liter
260 lbs	118 kg	16	130 oz	3.8 liter
280 lbs	127 kg	18	140 oz	4.1 liter
300 lbs	136 kg	19	150 oz	4.4 liter
320 lbs	145 kg	20	160 oz	4.7 liter

In addition to drinking water, consuming hydrating foods such as fruits and vegetables, and using moisturizers and skincare products containing hydrating ingredients can further support skin hydration and overall skin health. Regularly replenishing fluids and staying adequately hydrated can help promote radiant, supple, and healthy-looking skin. Drinking an adequate amount of water daily helps flush out toxins, improve skin elasticity, and keep the skin hydrated from within. For individuals who struggle with the taste of water, there are several strategies to increase water intake while still enjoying the experience:

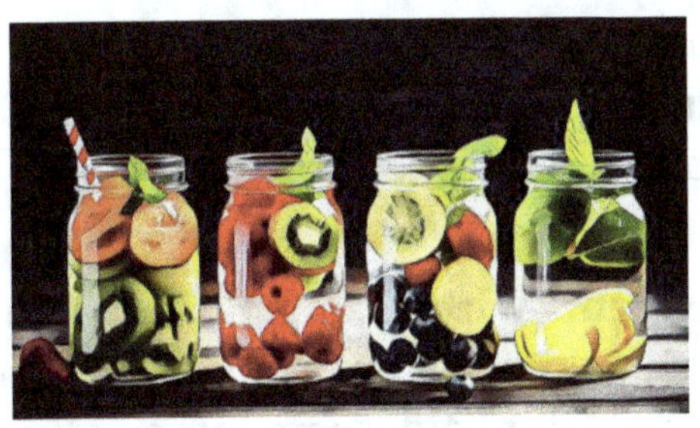

1. **Infuse Water with Fruits and Herbs:** Add slices of fruits like lemon, lime, orange, berries, or cucumber, along with fresh herbs like mint, basil, or rosemary, to a pitcher of water. This enhances the flavor of the water naturally and makes it more enjoyable to drink.

2. **Try Sparkling Water:** Sparkling water or carbonated water can provide a refreshing alternative to plain water. Look for unsweetened varieties to avoid added sugars and artificial flavors. You can also add a splash of fruit juice or a twist of citrus for extra flavor.

3. **Drink Herbal Tea:** Herbal teas, such as chamomile, peppermint, or fruit-infused blends, can be a hydrating and flavorful option for those who prefer warm beverages. Brew a pot of herbal tea and enjoy it hot or cold throughout the day.

4. **Consume Water-Rich Foods:** Incorporate water-rich foods into your diet, such as watermelon, cucumber, celery, oranges, and strawberries. These foods not only provide hydration but also add variety and flavor to your meals and snacks.

5. **Use Flavor Enhancers:** There are many flavor enhancers available in the market designed specifically for enhancing the taste of water. Look for natural flavor drops or water enhancers that are free from artificial sweeteners, colors, and preservatives.

6. **Set a Drinking Schedule:** Establish a drinking schedule

and aim to consume small amounts of water regularly throughout the day. This can help prevent dehydration and make it easier to incorporate more water into your daily routine.

7. **Experiment with Temperature:** Some people may prefer drinking water at different temperatures. Try drinking water cold, room temperature, or even warm to see which temperature you find most palatable.

By incorporating these strategies, individuals who dislike the taste of water can still meet their hydration needs while enjoying flavorful and refreshing alternatives.

Stress Management

Chronic stress can take a toll on skin health, leading to increased inflammation, breakouts, and accelerated aging. Practice stress management techniques such as mindfulness meditation, deep breathing exercises, or yoga to promote relaxation and reduce cortisol levels. Incorporating self-care activities like taking a warm bath, spending time in nature, or listening to soothing music can also help alleviate stress and improve overall well-being. Likewise, natural supplements such as ashwagandha has proven effective in regulating cortisol levels and sleep.

However, *individual responses to ashwagandha supplementation may vary, and it's always advisable to use caution. Do proper* *research and consult with a healthcare professional before incorporating any new supplement into your routine, **especially if you have underlying health conditions or are taking medications.***

Another method to reduce stress which has an anti-aging effect is called the Tanaka massage. The Tanaka massage, developed by Japanese 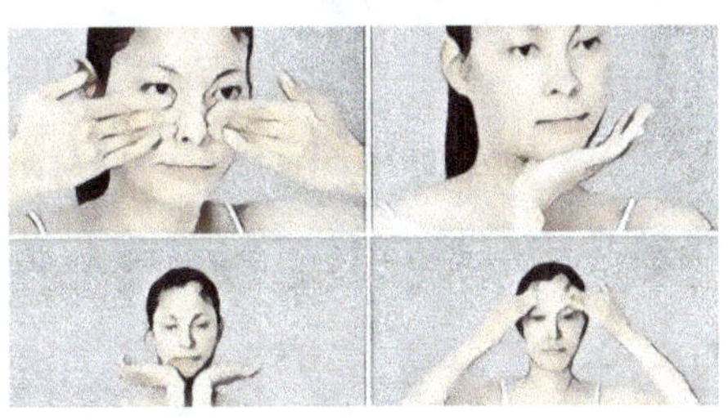 esthetician Yukuko Tanaka, is a facial massage technique renowned for its rejuvenating and anti-aging effects (improves skin elasticity, reduce puffiness, and diminish fine lines/wrinkles). This massage aids with stress regulation by incorporating techniques that promote relaxation and reduce tension in the facial muscles. During the massage, gentle, rhythmic motions are applied to various pressure points on the face, helping to release accumulated stress and tension. This massage also stimulates circulation and lymphatic drainage, which can help flush out toxins and reduce inflammation associated with stress.

As a result, the Tanaka massage induces a sense of calm and tranquility, helping to alleviate physical and mental stressors. The meditative and soothing nature of the massage further promotes relaxation, making it an effective tool for stress management and overall well-being.

Lymphatic System

Let's take a step back and delve into the specific role that the lymphatic system plays in promoting healthy skin. As mentioned earlier, the lymphatic system serves as a crucial mechanism for eliminating pathogens, toxins, and harmful substances from the body. It ensures that the pathway for delivering oxygen, nutrients, and hydration to the cells remains unobstructed and fully functional, which directly impacts the health and moisture balance of the skin. When the lymphatic system fails to function optimally or encounters obstacles in lymph flow, it can lead to various skin issues. These may include acne, decreased skin elasticity, premature aging, and a lackluster complexion characterized by dryness and flakiness.

Accumulation of toxins can cause the lymph to thicken, impeding its flow and disrupting the processes of cell renewal and repair. Blocked lymph flow can also result in cells being poisoned by their own waste, contributing to skin conditions such as acne, psoriasis, and eczema. This sluggish cycle of cell repair undermines efforts to achieve clear and healthy skin. Although it is often overlooked, ensuring the proper functioning of the lymphatic system is essential for maintaining skin health.

No worries, though. I bring good news. You're not stuck with a sluggish lymphatic system forever. There are some fun and effective ways to give it a boost and keep it in tip-top shape! A little love for your lymphatic system goes a long way toward achieving that radiant, glowing skin you've always envisioned. Remember: You are the superhero in your path to radiant skin. Six ways to ensure that your lymphatic system runs like a well-oiled machine are: exercise (walking, jogging, yoga), maintaining hydration, dry brushing, good posture, lymphatic massage, and facial exercises (see Tanaka massage).

Exercise And Sleep

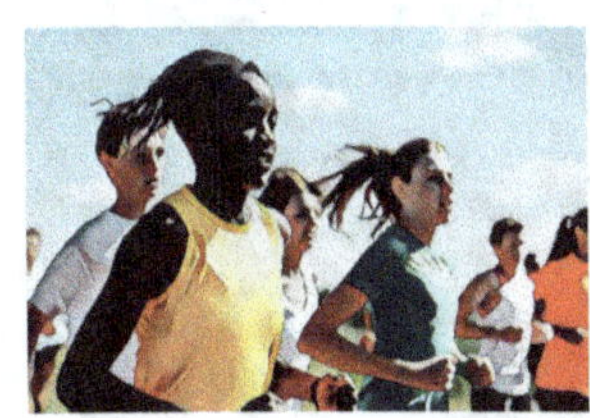

Regular physical activity not only benefits overall health but also plays a crucial role in skin health. Exercise increases blood flow, delivering oxygen and nutrients to the skin cells and promoting a healthy glow. Aim for at least 30 minutes of moderate-intensity exercise most days of the week to reap the skin-boosting benefits. For those who see exercise as thrilling as a trip to the dentist's chair, fear not! Besides the gym, here are some other activities that double as workouts.

1. Gardening or yard work
2. Dancing around the house while cleaning
3. Playing with pets, such as fetch or tug-of-war
4. Jumping on a trampoline
5. Hula hooping
6. Cleaning windows or washing the car by hand

7. Playing active video games, like Wii Fit or Dance Dance Revolution
8. Rollerblading or skateboarding
9. Rock climbing or bouldering
10. Indoor or outdoor obstacle courses

Additionally, prioritizing quality sleep is essential for skin repair and regeneration. Practice good sleep routine by establishing a consistent sleep schedule, creating a relaxing bedtime custom, and optimizing your sleep environment.

HOW MUCH SLEEP DO YOU NEED?

In 2015, a panel of experts in sleep, anatomy, physiology, pediatrics, neurology, gerontology and gynecology joined forces to create new, age-specific sleep recommendations.

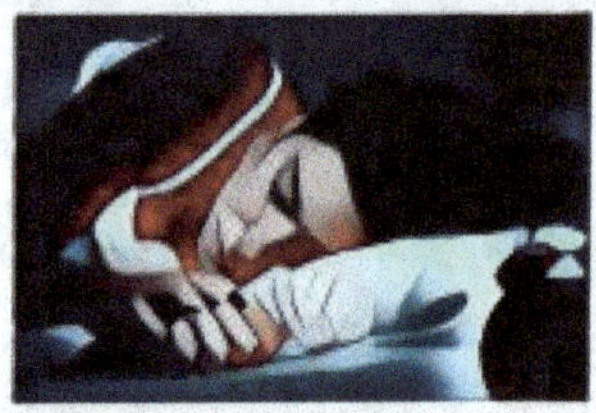

SLEEP TIMES ARE SHOWN ON A 24-HOUR CLOCK FACE

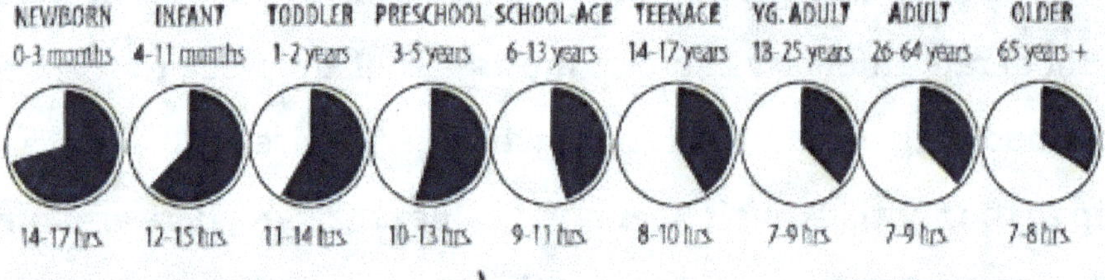

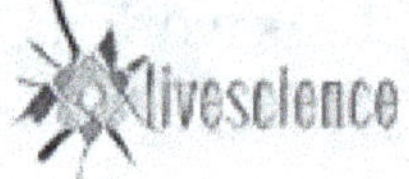

Poor sleep can have a significant impact on skin health, contributing to various skin issues and accelerating the aging process. Here are some ways in which inadequate sleep can affect the skin:

1. Increased Signs of Aging: During sleep, the body repairs and regenerates skin cells, producing collagen and elastin fibers essential for maintaining skin elasticity and firmness. Poor sleep disrupts this natural repair process, leading to a breakdown of collagen and elastin, which can result in the development of fine lines, wrinkles, and sagging skin (https://artofdermatology.com/how-sleep-affects-the-skin/).

2. Skin Dullness: Lack of sleep can cause poor blood circulation and reduce oxygen flow to the skin, resulting in a dull and lackluster complexion. Inadequate sleep also impairs the skin's ability to retain moisture, leading to dryness and flakiness.

3. Dark Circles and Puffiness: Insufficient sleep can cause fluid retention and blood vessels to dilate, leading to the appearance of dark circles and puffiness around the eyes. This occurs because poor sleep disrupts the body's natural fluid balance and lymphatic drainage system, resulting in fluid accumulation in the under-eye area.

4. Increased Skin Sensitivity: Lack of sleep can weaken the skin's protective barrier, making it more susceptible to environmental aggressors and irritants. This can lead to increased skin sensitivity, redness, and inflammation, exacerbating conditions like eczema, psoriasis, and acne.

5. Delayed Wound Healing: Adequate sleep is essential for proper wound healing and skin regeneration. Poor sleep can slow down the skin's ability to repair itself, prolonging the healing process for cuts, bruises, and other skin injuries.

Prioritizing quality sleep is essential for maintaining healthy, youthful-looking skin. Establishing a consistent sleep schedule, practicing good sleep hygiene habits, and addressing underlying sleep disorders can help support optimal skin health and function as well as overall wellbeing.

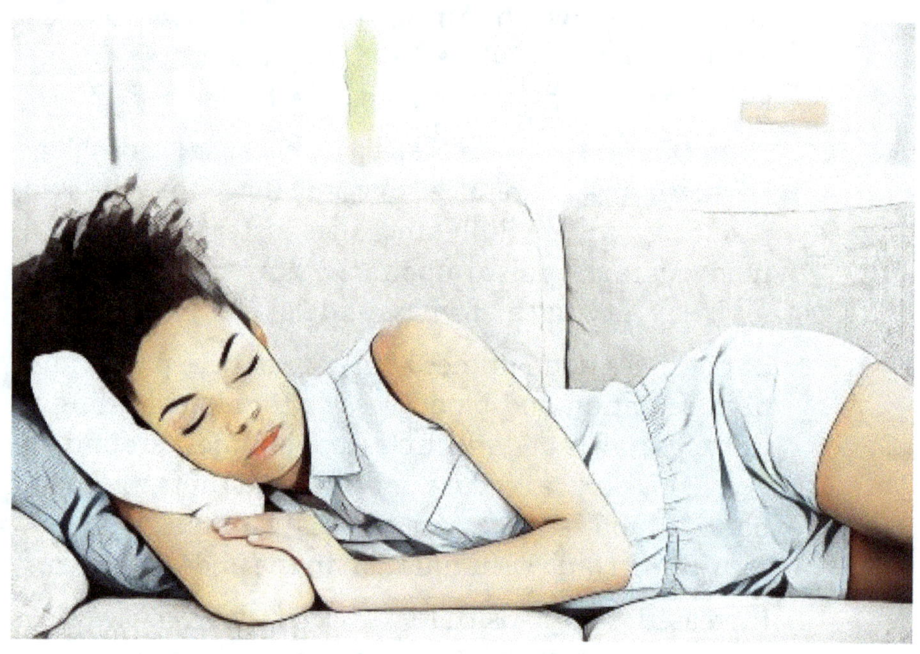

"SLEEP IS THE GOLDEN CHAIN THAT TIES HEALTH AND OUR BODIES TOGETHER." - THOMAS DEKKER

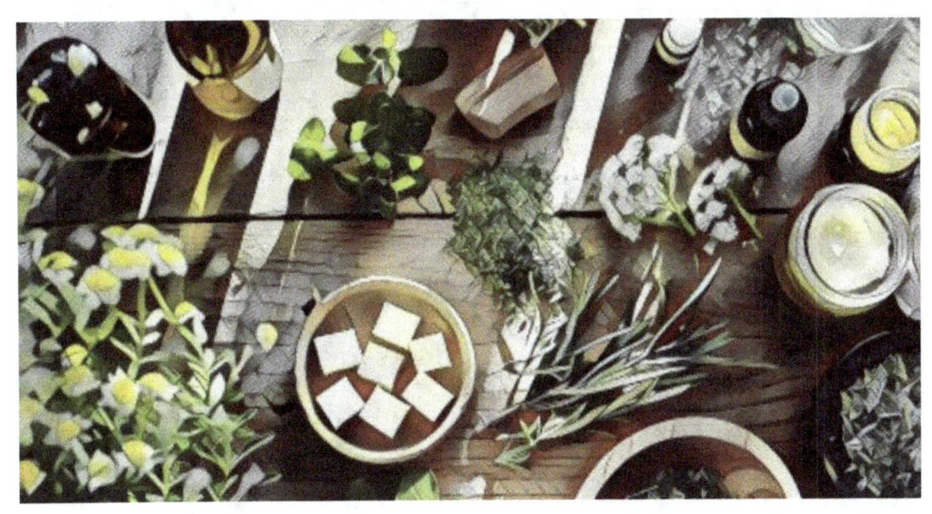

CHAPTER V:
REMEMBER THAT INGREDIENTS MATTER

Learn to read labels, not just for the fancy buzzwords but for the ingredients that actually matter. Retinoids, hyaluronic acid, niacinamide, and salicylic acid are not just industry jargon; they're proven ingredients that can significantly impact your skin's health. But remember, more is not always better. Overloading your skin with a cocktail of active ingredients can lead to irritation, sensitivity, and more problems than you started with.

You must still always remember that in a world inundated with chemical-laden skincare products, sometimes the most effective solutions are found in nature's embrace. Let's return to nature for the answer for a moment. Natural remedies offer a gentle yet potent approach to addressing stubborn facial skin problems, harnessing the power of botanical extracts, essential oils, and age-old remedies. These ingredients not only nourish and heal the skin but also minimize the risk of adverse reactions and environmental harm. Here are some natural remedies worth considering:

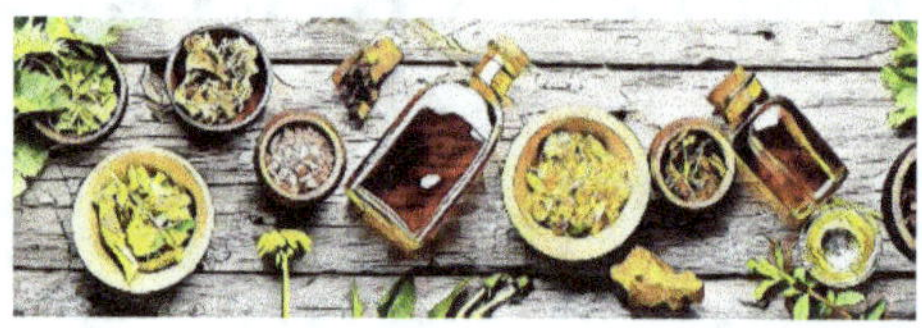

1. **Tea Tree Oil:** With its antimicrobial and anti-inflammatory properties, tea tree oil is a potent fighter against acne-causing bacteria. Dilute it with a carrier oil and apply it directly to blemishes for targeted treatment.

2. **Honey:** Nature's liquid gold, honey is renowned for its antibacterial and humectant properties. It moisturizes the skin while combating acne and soothing inflammation. Apply raw honey as a mask or spot treatment for a natural boost to your skincare routine.

3. **Aloe Vera:** This succulent plant is a skincare superhero, revered for its soothing, hydrating, and

healing properties. Aloe vera gel is particularly effective in calming irritated skin, reducing redness, and promoting healing.

4. **Castor Oil:** Castor oil is a true all-in-one skincare powerhouse, serving as a cleanser, skin firmer, healer, and moisturizer. Rich in ricinoleic acid, it boasts anti-inflammatory, antimicrobial, and moisturizing properties, making it suitable for a wide range of skin concerns.

   - As a cleanser, castor oil effectively dissolves impurities, excess oil, and makeup without stripping the skin's natural oils.

   - Its skin-firming properties help improve elasticity and tone, reducing the appearance of fine lines and wrinkles.

   - Castor oil's healing abilities make it ideal for soothing irritated or inflamed skin, including acne-prone or sunburned areas.

   - As a moisturizer, it penetrates deeply to hydrate and nourish the skin, leaving it soft, supple, and glowing.

To ensure thoroughness, here are the possible side effects of tea tree oil, honey, aloe vera, and castor oil.

1. **Tea Tree Oil:**
   - Skin Irritation: Some individuals may experience redness, itching, or irritation when tea tree oil is applied to the skin, especially if used undiluted.

   - Allergic Reactions: Rarely, tea tree oil may cause allergic reactions such as hives or rash in sensitive individuals.

   - Eye Irritation: Direct contact with tea tree oil

can cause irritation to the eyes, leading to redness, stinging, or tearing.

2. **Honey:**

- Allergic Reactions: Although rare, some people may be allergic to honey, resulting in symptoms such as itching, swelling, or hives.

- Stickiness: Honey can be sticky and may cause discomfort if not thoroughly washed off the skin, particularly in humid climates or if left on for extended periods.

3. **Aloe Vera:**

- Skin Irritation: In some cases, aloe vera may cause skin irritation, especially in individuals with sensitive skin or allergies.

- Photosensitivity: Aloe vera gel may increase the skin's sensitivity to sunlight, leading to sunburn or skin reactions if exposed to UV rays without proper sun protection.

4. **Castor Oil:**

- Skin Irritation: Castor oil is generally considered safe for most people, but in some individuals, it may cause mild irritation or allergic reactions.

- Pore Clogging: Due to its thick consistency, castor oil may clog pores in some people, leading to breakouts or acne if not properly removed from the skin.

- Digestive Issues: When taken orally, castor oil may cause gastrointestinal discomfort, cramping, or diarrhea in some individuals.

Diy Recipes

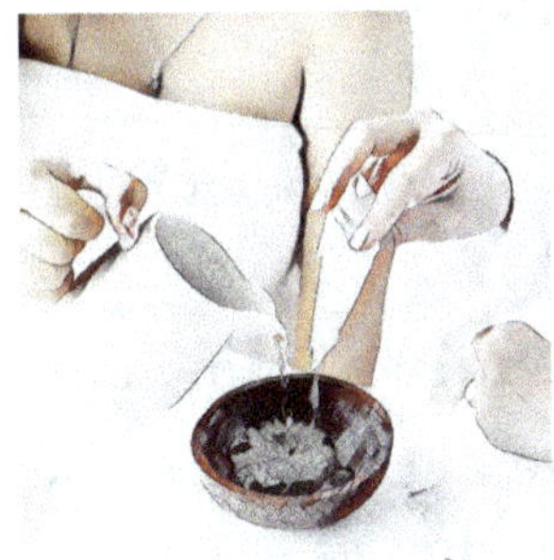

In case you're feeling more daring and hands-on with your skincare, get ready to unleash your inner skincare chef and embark on a DIY adventure that'll make your skin sing with joy! These recipes are akin to concoctions crafted by a skincare expert (that's you!) using ingredients sourced from a bountiful garden. Picture yourself as a skincare whiz, creating elixirs that'll have your skin glowing so bright, it'll outshine the sun! So put on your apron and let's dive into these recipes that'll make your skin happier than a unicorn at a glitter party!

1. **Honey and Oatmeal Face Mask:**
   - Ingredients:
     - 2 tablespoons oatmeal (ground into a fine powder)
     - 1 tablespoon honey
     - 1 tablespoon plain yogurt
   - Instructions:
     - Mix all ingredients together in a bowl until well combined.
     - Apply the mixture to clean, damp skin and leave on for 15-20 minutes.
     - Rinse off with warm water and pat dry. Follow with your favorite moisturizer.

2. **Avocado and Honey Moisturizing Mask:**
   - Ingredients:
     - 1 ripe avocado

- 1 tablespoon honey
- Instructions:
  - Mash the avocado in a bowl until smooth.
  - Stir in the honey until well combined.
  - Apply the mixture to clean skin and leave on for 15-20 minutes.
  - Rinse off with lukewarm water and gently pat dry.

3. **Yogurt and Turmeric Brightening Mask:**
   - Ingredients:
     - 2 tablespoons plain yogurt
     - 1/2 teaspoon turmeric powder
     - 1 teaspoon honey (optional)
   - Instructions:
     - Mix the yogurt and turmeric powder together in a bowl.
     - Add honey if desired for extra hydration.
     - Apply the mixture to cleansed skin and leave on for 10-15 minutes.
     - Rinse off with cool water and follow with moisturizer.

4. **Coconut Oil and Brown Sugar Scrub:**
   - Ingredients:
     - 2 tablespoons coconut oil (melted)
     - 2 tablespoons brown sugar
   - Instructions:
     - Mix the coconut oil and brown sugar together in a bowl until well

combined.

- Gently massage the mixture onto damp skin using circular motions for 2-3 minutes.

- Rinse off with warm water and pat dry. Follow with moisturizer for soft, smooth skin.

Here Are Some Bonus Diy Recipes With Included Benefits.

Soothing Palmarosa Oil Face Mask:

Ingredients:

1 tablespoon Plain Yogurt

1 teaspoon Honey

2-3 drops Palmarosa Essential Oil

Directions:

In a small bowl, mix together the plain yogurt and honey until well combined.

Add 2-3 drops of palmarosa essential oil to the mixture and stir thoroughly.

Cleanse your face with a gentle cleanser and pat dry.

Apply the mask evenly to your face, avoiding the delicate eye area.

Relax and leave the mask on for 10-15 minutes to allow the soothing properties of the ingredients to work their magic.

After the allotted time, rinse off the mask with lukewarm water and gently pat your skin dry.

Follow up with your favorite moisturizer to lock in hydration.

Benefits:

Yogurt: Yogurt contains lactic acid, which helps exfoliate dead skin cells and promote skin renewal. It also has soothing properties that can calm irritated skin and reduce redness.

Honey: Honey is a natural humectant, meaning it draws moisture into the skin, helping to hydrate and soothe dry, irritated skin. It also has antimicrobial properties that can help prevent infection and promote healing.

Palmarosa Essential Oil: Palmarosa oil has calming and soothing properties that can help reduce inflammation and irritation. It also has antibacterial and antifungal properties, making it beneficial for maintaining a healthy skin barrier.

This soothing palmarosa oil face mask is gentle yet effective, making it suitable for all skin types, especially those prone to irritation or sensitivity. Incorporate it into your skincare routine as needed to help calm and comfort irritated skin, leaving it feeling soft, smooth, and refreshed.

Hydrating Facial Serum:

Ingredients:

1 tablespoon Marula Oil

4 drops Geranium Oil

4 drops Palmarosa Oil

Directions:

In a small glass bottle, combine the marula oil with the geranium and palmarosa oils.

Gently shake the bottle to mix the ingredients thoroughly.

After cleansing your face, apply a few drops of the serum to damp skin and massage it in using upward circular motions.

Allow the serum to absorb fully before applying moisturizer.

Benefits:

Marula oil deeply moisturizes the skin, leaving it soft and supple.

Geranium oil helps balance sebum production and promotes clear, healthy-looking skin.

Palmarosa oil has antibacterial properties and helps maintain skin's moisture balance, reducing the risk of breakouts.

Rosehip Oil Facial Serum

Ingredients:

- 1 tablespoon rosehip oil
- 2-3 drops lavender essential oil
- 2-3 drops frankincense essential oil

Instructions:

1. In a small glass bottle, mix together the rosehip oil, lavender essential oil, and frankincense essential oil.
2. Close the bottle tightly and shake well to blend the oils.
3. After cleansing your face, apply a few drops of the serum onto your fingertips.
4. Gently massage the serum onto your face and neck using upward circular motions until fully absorbed.
5. Allow the serum to penetrate your skin for a few minutes before applying moisturizer or sunscreen.

Benefits:

- Rosehip oil is rich in antioxidants and essential fatty acids, which help hydrate and nourish the skin.
- Lavender essential oil has soothing properties that can calm irritated skin and promote relaxation.
- Frankincense essential oil is known for its anti-aging benefits and can help improve skin tone and texture.

This DIY facial serum is suitable for all skin types and can be used daily to promote healthy, radiant skin.

It's essential to perform a patch test before using these ingredients, _**especially if you have sensitive skin or known allergies. If you experience any adverse reactions, discontinue use immediately and consult a healthcare professional.**_ Overall, incorporating natural remedies like castor oil into your skincare routine not only promotes healthier skin but also aligns with a more sustainable and eco-conscious approach to beauty. Let's harness the power of nature to unlock the secrets of radiant, resilient skin.

Consistency Is Key

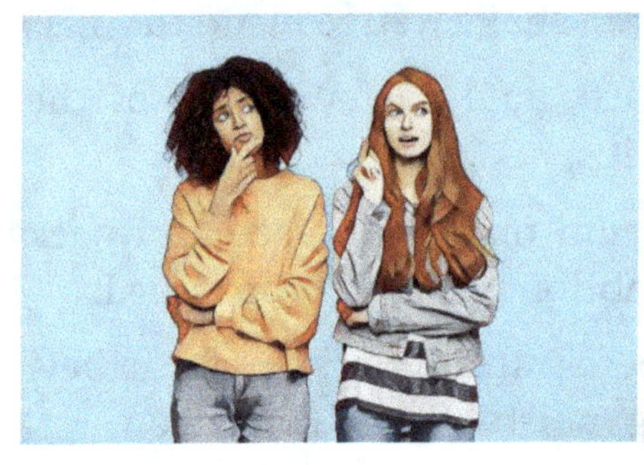

Perhaps the bluntest advice I can offer is this: skincare is a marathon, not a sprint. Results take time, patience, and consistency. Jumping from product to product in search of a quick fix often leads to frustration and wasted money. Yes, I'm talking about you… who want everything to work within the blink of an eye. Alright, let's pause with that skeptical side eye for a hot minute…or maybe two, or just make it three. Find what works for you and stick with it. Give it time to work its magic. Then, the magic will work for you. Remember, patience is a virtue. Chapter VI has a handy tool to aid in your skincare journey.

The Bottom Line

The path to solving stubborn facial skin problems is as much about what you avoid as what you embrace. Steer clear of unrealistic promises, understand the basics, and be willing to adjust your approach as you learn more about what your skin truly needs. Always be open to discovering a new path to an old problem, because the journey to healthier skin is a personal one, full of learning, patience, and, most importantly, self-love.

Embark on the quest for radiant skin like a skincare warrior, armed with moisturizers and serums instead of swords. Dodge the pitfalls of unrealistic promises and embrace the simplicity of the basics. Remember, the journey to healthier skin is like a rollercoaster ride - full of twists, turns, and occasional screams, but ultimately worth it for the selfie-worthy glow waiting at the end.

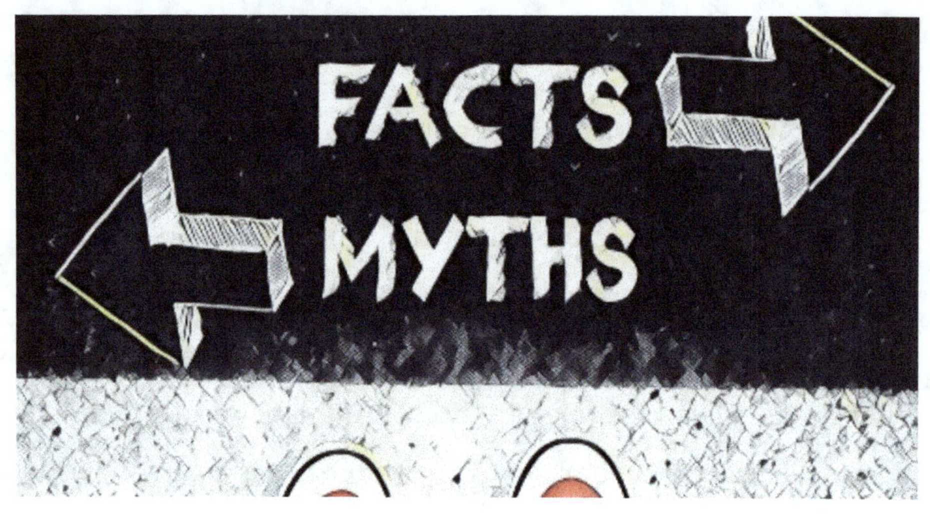

CHAPTER VI: MYTH-BUSTING AND FAQS

In this chapter, we'll address common myths surrounding skincare and provide answers to frequently asked questions related to skin health and maintenance.

Addressing Common Myths:

1. *Myth: Moisturizing Causes Acne.*
   Fact: Contrary to popular belief, moisturizing is essential for all skin types, including oily and acne-prone skin. Using a non-comedogenic moisturizer helps maintain the skin's moisture balance without clogging pores or exacerbating acne.

I hear ya, I hear ya! It's been written enough. You're probably

scratching your head and thinking, "What in tarnation does non-comedogenic even mean?"

A non-comedogenic moisturizer is a skincare product formulated with ingredients that are less likely to clog pores and cause acne breakouts. The term "comedogenic" refers to substances that have the potential to block or congest pores, leading to the formation of comedones (commonly known as blackheads and whiteheads) and other types of acne.

Non-comedogenic moisturizers are specifically designed to provide hydration and nourishment to the skin without exacerbating acne or contributing to pore congestion. These moisturizers typically contain lightweight, oil-free formulations that absorb easily into the skin without leaving a greasy or heavy residue.

Key characteristics of non-comedogenic moisturizers include:

> ***Oil-Free Formulation:*** *Non-comedogenic moisturizers are often oil-free or contain lightweight, non-greasy oils that are less likely to clog pores, such as jojoba oil or squalane.*

> ***Hypoallergenic Ingredients:*** *These moisturizers are formulated with hypoallergenic ingredients that are less likely to cause allergic reactions or irritate sensitive skin.*

> ***Non-Comedogenic Ingredients:*** *Non-comedogenic moisturizers typically contain ingredients that have a low comedogenic rating, meaning they are less likely to block pores and contribute to acne formation. Common non-comedogenic ingredients include glycerin, hyaluronic acid, and ceramides.*

> ***Fragrance-Free:*** *Fragrances can sometimes irritate*

the skin and exacerbate acne, so non-comedogenic moisturizers are often fragrance-free or contain minimal fragrance to reduce the risk of sensitivity reactions.

Overall, non-comedogenic moisturizers are suitable for individuals with acne-prone or oily skin types who are looking for lightweight hydration without the risk of pore congestion or breakouts. These moisturizers provide essential moisture to the skin while helping to maintain a clear and healthy complexion.

2. *Myth: Sunscreen Is Only Necessary on Sunny Days.*
   Fact: Sunscreen should be applied daily, regardless of the weather. UV rays can penetrate through clouds and windows, leading to sun damage and premature aging. Incorporating sunscreen into your daily skincare routine helps protect the skin from harmful UV radiation.

3. *Myth: Natural Ingredients Are Always Better for the Skin.*
   Fact: While natural ingredients offer numerous skincare benefits, not all natural ingredients are suitable for every skin type. It's essential to consider factors such as skin sensitivities and allergies when choosing skincare products, whether they contain natural or synthetic ingredients.

If you believe in the power of notation like me, allow me to introduce the Skin Diary, your trusty sidekick in the quest for radiant skin! It's time to grab your pen or fire up that digital device and start documenting your skincare journey. With this handy diary, you can track every step of your routine, from cleansing to moisturizing and beyond. Keep tabs on the products you're using and how your skin responds to them. Is that new serum giving you that coveted glow, or is it causing a breakout that rivals Mount

Vesuvius? Only one way to find out! Plus, this diary includes prompts to help you jot down observations about changes in your skin texture, hydration levels, and any pesky blemishes that dare to make an appearance. So, let's get journaling and uncover the secrets to your best skin ever!

Skin Diary

Date: _________________________

Morning Routine:

1. **Cleanser:** _________________________
   - How does your skin feel after cleansing? _________________________

2. **Toner:** _________________________
   - Any changes in skin texture or appearance? _________________________

3. **Serum:** _________________________
   - Notice any improvements or changes in hydration levels? _________________________

4. **Moisturizer:** _________________________
   - Is your skin feeling adequately hydrated? _________________________

5. **Sunscreen:** _________________________
   - Any reactions or changes in skin condition after applying sunscreen? _________________________

Evening Routine:

1. **Makeup Remover/Cleansing:** _________________________
   - How effectively did it remove makeup and impurities? _________________________

2. **Exfoliant (if applicable):** ______________________
    - Any changes in skin texture or clarity? ______________________

3. **Toner:** ______________________
    - Did it leave your skin feeling balanced and refreshed? ______________________

4. **Treatment (if applicable):** ______________________
    - Any noticeable improvements in specific skin concerns? ______________________

5. **Moisturizer:** ______________________
    - Is your skin feeling nourished and hydrated? ______________________

Additional Notes:

- **Diet:** Any changes in diet or hydration levels that may affect skin health? ______________________

- **Sleep:** How many hours of sleep did you get last night? Any noticeable impact on skin condition? ______________________

- **Stress Levels:** Rate your stress levels on a scale of 1 to 10. Any correlation with changes in skin? ______________________

- **Overall Skin Condition:** Describe how your skin feels and looks today. Any specific concerns or improvements? ______________________

Feel free to print and use this skin diary to track your skincare routine and monitor changes in your skin over time. Happy journaling!

Answering Frequently Asked Questions:

1. *FAQ: How Often Should I Exfoliate My Skin?*
   Answer: The frequency of exfoliation depends on your skin type and the type of exfoliant used. For most people, exfoliating 2-3 times per week is sufficient to remove dead skin cells and promote cell turnover. However, individuals with sensitive or acne-prone skin may benefit from less frequent exfoliation to avoid irritation.

2. *FAQ: Can I Use Retinol and Vitamin C Together?*
   Answer: Yes, retinol and vitamin C can be used together in a skincare routine. Both ingredients offer unique benefits for the skin, with retinol promoting cell turnover and collagen production, while vitamin C provides antioxidant protection and brightening effects. To minimize the risk of irritation, start by using each ingredient on alternate nights and gradually increase frequency as tolerated.

3. *FAQ: What Should I Do If I Have a Skincare Reaction?*
   Answer: If you experience a skincare reaction such as redness, itching, or irritation, immediately stop using the product that caused the reaction. Rinse your face with water to remove any remaining product and apply a soothing, gentle moisturizer to calm the skin. If the reaction persists or worsens, consult a dermatologist for further evaluation and treatment.

By debunking common skincare myths and providing answers to frequently asked questions, I hope to empower you with accurate information to achieve healthier, happier skin. As we conclude this journey together, remember that your skin health is an ongoing process, and every step you take towards caring for it matters. Armed with the knowledge and tools provided in this e-book, you have the power to transform your skincare routine and achieve radiant, healthy skin. Embrace consistency. Listen to your skin's needs, and don't hesitate to seek professional advice when necessary. Your skin is unique, beautiful, and deserving of the best care. Here's to your continued journey towards glowing skin and newfound confidence. My final thought I leave with you is beauty begins within and stay the course. Thank you for allowing me to be a part of it.

Chapter I quiz results

Results:

Mostly A's: You likely have normal skin, which is well-balanced and not overly oily or dry.

Mostly B's: Your skin may be combination, with oilier areas in the T-zone and drier patches elsewhere.

Mostly C's: You may have oily or acne-prone skin, with excess oil production and a tendency to develop blemishes.

Mostly D's: Your skin may be dry or sensitive, with a tendency to feel tight, flaky, or irritated.

ABOUT THE AUTHOR

Mechiebee

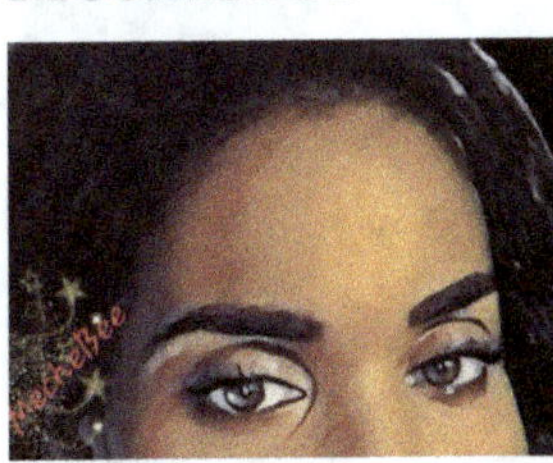

I'm a passionate lady who has embarked on countless skincare journeys, experimenting with a myriad of products along the way. Through my experiences, I have come to understand that each skincare journey is a deeply personal, yet undeniably rewarding and fulfilling. Through keen observation, commitment, and joy to share my insights, I want to help others to be daring and embrace their unique paths to radiant skin. Join me in the continual discovery in this intricate world of skincare.